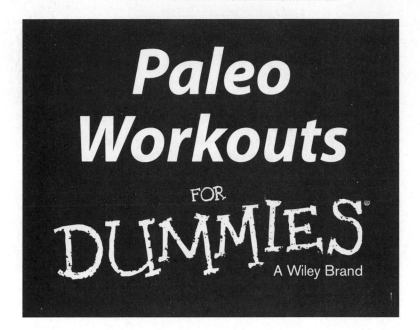

Paleo Workouts

FOR DUMMIES

A Wiley Brand

by Dr. Kellyann Petrucci and Patrick Flynn

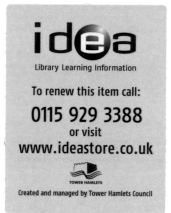
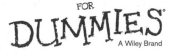

FOR
DUMMIES
A Wiley Brand

Paleo Workouts For Dummies®

Published by: **John Wiley & Sons, Inc.,** 111 River Street, Hoboken, NJ 07030-5774, www.wiley.com

For general information on our other products and services, please contact our Customer Care Department within the U.S. at 877-762-2974, outside the U.S. at 317-572-3993, or fax 317-572-4002. For technical support, please visit www.wiley.com/techsupport.

Wiley publishes in a variety of print and electronic formats and by print-on-demand. Some material included with standard print versions of this book may not be included in e-books or in print-on-demand. If this book refers to media such as a CD or DVD that is not included in the version you purchased, you may download this material at http://booksupport.wiley.com. For more information about Wiley products, visit www.wiley.com.

Library of Congress Control Number: 2013949062

ISBN 978-1-118-65791-1 (pbk); ISBN 978-1-118-75593-8 (ebk); ISBN 978-1-118-75595-2 (ebk); ISBN 978-1-118-75607-2 (ebk)

Manufactured in the United States of America

10 9 8 7 6 5 4 3 2 1

Contents at a Glance

Table of Contents

Introduction

∙ ∙

*D*on't expect to find anything new and exciting in this book because whenever someone comes along with a "new and exciting" exercise program, it's generally all wrong. When it comes to fitness, a new way of doing something is rarely a better way of doing something. It's almost invariably the exchange of one nuisance for another.

Everything people need to know about fitness is already known. And everything people need to do, they can already do. Getting lean, fit, healthy, and strong aren't functions of addition but rather subtraction. It's a matter of scaling back — separating the gold from the garbage — and focusing on the vital few efforts that are proven to get you the best results.

Paleo Workouts For Dummies is about scaling back and reducing exercise to its lowest, most profitable efforts. In other words, it's about exercising like a cave man: no fancy equipment required — just big, beautiful movements.

About This Book

A big part of *Paleo Workouts For Dummies* is dedicated to movement. Movement needs to be taken seriously. Movement *is* life after all; the old and dying are always stiff and hard, whereas the young and healthy are soft and supple. Age is but a number, friends. You are only as old as how well you move.

In this book, we help you move better by providing step-by-step tutorials on how to move more athletically, naturally. We provide the tips and tricks you need to move and exercise with near faultless form so you stay free from injury and get the most out of the exercise programs in Part III.

This book is also about helping you exercise more deliberately, or with a purpose. We provide specific, primal exercise programs designed to transform your body. When we say *primal,* we mean that all the exercise programs are centered on the fundamental human movements — pushing, pulling, hinging, squatting, and carrying — the movements that burn the most calories and build the most muscle.

Just as the Paleo diet is about eating like our ancestors (which we talk about in Part IV of this book), Paleo fitness is about moving like them. This means heavy lifting, sprinting, brisk walking, and a few other movements that the conveniences of modern day have made largely irrelevant.

This book is a stark movement in the opposite direction of the masses. It's unconventional, it's contrarian, and it's effective. And we say without any reservations whatsoever that if you truly want to blast fat, boost muscle, and build resilience, well, this book may be one of the most important books you ever read.

Foolish Assumptions

We assume only one thing about you, and that is that you want to improve your general condition or perhaps one condition specifically. We make that general assumption based on the following ideas about you, dear reader:

- You want to be healthier, leaner, stronger, or more productive. Or perhaps you want to be all these things.
- You want to lose weight, increase lean muscle mass, and improve athletic performance.
- You don't know much about Paleo fitness.
- You've tried exercise programs in the past and haven't been satisfied with the results or have been frustrated with the process.
- You have your doctor's approval to do the exercise programs in this book.

   Note: We recommend that you get your doctor's approval before beginning any exercise program, whether you're a novice or a veteran to fitness.

Icons Used in This Book

Throughout this book, and in true *For Dummies* fashion, you'll see a number of icons in the margins — all of them designed to help you better understand and get the most out of your Paleo fitness journey. Here are the icons and what each one means.

This icon highlights info that will help you better understand a concept or help you put a concept into action.

This icon points out any information we deem important to remember as you adapt to Paleo living.

We don't post warnings often, but when we do, pay attention, because they're important. Don't skip over these icons, less you want to fall into a potentially harmful mistake!

This icon flags the nitty-gritty and often scientific details about certain concepts. This information is optional but certainly recommended!

Beyond the Book

We think this book is a great resource for getting healthy, lean, and strong. But there's way more to this book than just what you can find in the text. We provide a bunch of additional information on Dummies.com:

- ✔ You can download the book's Cheat Sheet at www.dummies.com/cheatsheet/paleoworkouts. It's a handy resource to keep on your computer, tablet, or smartphone.

- ✔ Coauthor Pat Flynn demonstrates dozens of exercises that are featured in the book. You can see the videos and explore more aspects of the Paleo lifestyle at www.dummies.com/go/paleo.

- ✔ You can read interesting companion articles that supplement the book's content at www.dummies.com/extras/paleoworkouts. We've even written an extra top-ten list.

Where to Go from Here

In short, read Part I to understand what Paleo fitness is all about. Then go to Parts II and III to begin exercising. Part IV gets you started on Paleo nutrition. Jump around as you see fit, or read the book from front to back. It's up to you.

We ask you to proceed only with an open mind. Much of what you're about to read is in stark opposition to conventional wisdom. And because of that, some of the practices in this book remain controversial. But remember this statement from Mark Twain: "Whenever you find yourself on the side of the majority, it's time to pause and reflect."

Also, conventional wisdom has failed quite miserably, hasn't it? The United States and much of the Western world are dealing with perhaps the worst health crisis the world has ever known. People are fatter and unhealthier than ever. The prevalence of diabetes, cancer, and heart disease is alarming.

Yet no one's waking up. The junk people eat and their sedentary lifestyle have created a population that's more sick than healthy. This is not how it's supposed to be. Humans are meant to be both vibrant and resilient. We're meant to move. Now get moving!

Part I

Getting Started with Paleo Fitness

getting started with

paleo

fitness

Visit www.dummies.com for more great Dummies content online.

In this part . . .

- ✔ Discover why paring down an exercise program to its most essential parts will garner you greater fitness success than following mainstream programs that believe in a "more is better" policy.

- ✔ Find out why the kettlebell may just be the most perfect tool when it comes to the Paleo fitness style of training.

- ✔ Recognize how seemingly simple things, such as breathing, daily movement, and fasting, can have profound and lasting effects on your fitness, health, and overall wellness.

- ✔ Understand why the Paleo diet — a diet in which you cut out grains, refined sugars, dairy, and legumes, among other things — is a perfect complement to the Paleo fitness lifestyle and how combining the two can catapult your results.

- ✔ Master the three primal movements that everyone should be able to perform and find out why these exercises are imperative to your health.

Chapter 1

Paleo Fitness: The (Ab)Original Blueprint for Physical Excellence

In This Chapter

▶ Changing your mindset to Paleo fitness

▶ Comparing Paleo fitness to conventional programs

▶ Following the cave man's way of health and fitness

▶ Seeing (and feeling) results with Paleo

▶ Getting started with Paleo fitness

*1*t's been quite some time since the public was afforded the luxury of an exercise program that actually makes sense and isn't full of absurdities or ridiculousness. From diet pills to shake weights, "progress" in terms of health and fitness over the past decade has been little more than the swapping of one gimmick for another.

Paleo fitness is not about presenting something new; it's about getting back to what works. Because we already know what works, and we always have.

Paleo fitness means working out like a cave man. We use the cave man to symbolize the idea of getting back to basics, specifically in these areas:

✔ Back to the big, fundamental human movements

✔ Back to movement that is beautiful, unrestricted, and pain-free

✔ Back to movements proven effective for burning fat, building muscle, and boosting resilience

So we want you to perform all movements that the cave man needed to do on a daily basis to survive. And that means pushing, pulling, hinging, squatting, sprinting, carrying, and jumping.

Shifting Your Paradigm to Paleo: Live Long, Live Strong

Most people think that bodily health is plainly the result of eating less of what they want to eat and doing more of the things they don't want to do. But we aim to challenge that assumption to prove that a beautiful body and beautiful movement can be the result of an enjoyable, active lifestyle and not grunting and tears.

When you first change your paradigm to Paleo fitness, it may feel a little odd, and that's okay. In a world of "more, more, more," doing less often feels weird. And at times on this Paleo journey, you'll feel like you haven't even worked out at all. Not a bead of sweat will drop from your brow. You'll be done with your workout in less than 15 minutes, and that'll be it for the day.

You may even feel almost as if you're cheating. And perhaps, in a way, you are cheating because, perhaps, you have a slightly unfair advantage. That advantage is knowledge — the ability to understand that working out isn't all about the sweat or the burn. And knowing that *effort* isn't synonymous with *effective;* in other words, *working hard* doesn't always mean *working right*.

Changing your mindset to Paleo is tough at first. The primal aficionado sometimes feels like an outcast, like a kid at the adult dinner table. But before you think it's too much, think on this: Your health is like a balance sheet. Everything you do — every single choice you make — is debited or credited; it either improves your position or worsens it. And your health, to put it simply, is nothing more than the accrual of all the decisions you've ever made.

What we're saying here is that health is a choice. Strength is a choice, too. And your job is to do everything you possibly can to continuously improve your position.

The Paleo community has a mantra: "Live long. Drop dead." The implication of this statement is that as long as you live in accordance to the blueprint set forth by our ancestors, then you live a life relatively free of ailments. We add the phrase "live strong" to this mantra for two reasons: (1) We find that strong people, as Greg Glassman once so eloquently put it, are "generally more useful than weak people," and (2) they are, without question, quite harder to kill.

Paleo Fitness: Discovering the Difference

Most conventional dietary and fitness plans are conspiracies against mankind. They offer little in the way of reasonableness or sustainability and are largely set to fail from the start. But Paleo has changed the game by going in the opposite direction. And the Paleo diet has become nothing short of a welcome phenomenon, helping hundreds of thousands of people all over the world lose weight and restore health. As you discover throughout this book, Paleo fitness works in much the same way. It reverse-engineers the habits of the proverbial cave man and makes them applicable to modern life.

We've taken the brakes off success simply by reversing direction. Now you, too, can quickly achieve optimal health, strength, and vitality when you mimic the physical behavior of our ancestors — our way, way back ancestors, that is.

Paleo fitness success story: Peter

Meet Peter, 24, security officer; Oshkosh, Wisconsin:

As a lifetime athlete, Peter used to rest on the belief that he could compensate for a somewhat questionable diet through massive caloric burns in practice and competitive environments through grade school and high school. When Peter got into his college football career at the University of Wisconsin-Oshkosh, he sustained a major concussion early in his sophomore year. Not being able to work out because of the injury paired with a feeling of deep depression, he turned to pizza, cake, and doughnuts to help him cope with the pain, but these choices were harming him more than helping him. Having prolonged symptoms from his head injury stretch out beyond six months, Peter's weight ballooned up close to the 390-pound mark. When Peter thought he finally felt better, he attempted a light workout only to have extreme feelings of vertigo and a sharp pain where his spine met his brain stem. After some reoccurrence of this feeling, he sought the medical advice of numerous doctors who all told him the same thing: His bad cholesterol paired with high blood pressure brought him mere seconds away from having a stroke if he would have continued to exert himself, and Peter was only 21 years old!

Being utterly shaken by this news from the doctors, Peter decided he was going to wise up. And it was around this time that Peter discovered Paleo fitness, introduced to him by a close friend. He began walking long distances until he could begin to jog, and then Peter began to run and sprint short distances. He began to pay far more attention to not only how his body was reacting to subtle changes of movement but also how he fueled his body. Peter instantly noticed a change when he began ingesting wholesome, Paleo foods and followed a Paleo fitness regimen. What surprised Peter the most was that with very simple, conscientious changes in his lifestyle, the weight simply fell off in mass.

Paleo fitness has led Peter to some truly amazing outcomes and milestones along his journey to full body health and wellness. Peter has lost more than 120 pounds and is feeling healthier than ever! What Peter has been most proud of, however, are the strength gains he has made over the course of the journey. The Paleo fitness lifestyle has also led Peter to develop the overall fitness level necessary to excel in physical fitness testing for police departments in his home state of Wisconsin.

Paleo fitness is just as old as it is new. You can discover everything you need to know about how to achieve the body of your dreams by looking at the lifestyle of our Paleolithic ancestors.

With few exceptions, all progress in the realm of fitness since the era of the cave man hasn't really been progress at all. People have added many nuisances and plenty of distractions in the past 2.6 million years, no doubt, but few true advances.

In fact, humans are the unhealthiest and fattest they've ever been. And sadly, this steady rise in obesity has convinced some scientists to suggest that we may experience, for the first time in history, a decline in life expectancy in the 21st century. Does this surprise you?

Opinions on effective solutions to this problem vary, seemingly, by year. But the truth is that everything that could ever be known on how to live a strong and healthy life is already known — that is, we already know what we need to do to live a long and healthy life based on how our ancestors lived. Any distinct contributions made since then and henceforth amount to very little.

Humans are naturally designed to be strong and healthy. So to look, feel, and perform your best, you have to do the things you were designed to do. This book lays it all out for you.

Patterning Life after the Cave Man

The cave man was perhaps a perfect role model for health and exercise because he didn't try to improve something that was virtually faultless. He followed his genetic programming: He moved how he was meant to move and ate how he was meant to eat. He was fit and healthy.

In the domain of exercise today, fads come (and just as often go) like pimples on a teenybopper. Most of these crazes are, at best, useless, but quite a few have even grown to be dangerous, which concerns us. Our concern lies in not only poor movement but also the gross lack of desire, or priority, for strong, beautiful movement.

Only a handful of popular fitness practices approach exercise this way. Most make people move but fail to first show them how to do so. Many fitness programs make the conventional assumption that people just know how to move, or that they know how to move well. However, for most, quality movement is like writing cursive — an elegant skill that gets sloppy without practice.

Too many people don't give enough respect to strong, beautiful movement. We admit, however, that although most conventional fitness fashions neglect strength and movement quality, they do serve a hidden but useful purpose: They remind people of our values and why this book is important.

In the following sections, we introduce these values in the form of principles as they pertain to Paleo fitness and how they can help you achieve a leaner, harder, and more resilient physique. Understand that many of these principles directly contradict conventional fitness practices — that's the point.

Conditioning yourself for something other than exercise

The first principle of Paleo fitness states that the most basic and appropriate function of exercise should be to condition someone for something other than exercise. Whether that something is a sport is of small significance. Exercise is, and should remain, a means (a method) to an end (a goal), but many conventional fitness practices forget this detail, because they take the means (exercise) and make it an ends (a sport or competition).

Exercise should be a means to health. Exercise should promote health and vitality — and never, under any circumstance, should it ever detract from that. When that is covered, you may then explore exercise as a means to other ends, such as for spiritual purposes or athletic enhancement.

The harm comes when people turn exercise into a competitive sport. Quality is swapped for quantity, and people get hurt. Exercise should make you better at all things, at all times, and in every way. Anything else simply won't do.

Getting just the right amount of exercise

The second principle of Paleo fitness states that exercise is best served in small to moderate doses, which is to say just enough to get the job done and not a smidgeon more. But again, conventional practices overlook this detail, made clear by the number of people who spend hours every day trudging on treadmills and spinning on bicycles. Practices that create a chronic state of stress on the body are ill suited for sustainable bodily profits, not to mention wholly ineffective for long-term weight loss. Again, exercise should make you better at all things, at all times, and in every way.

Now the "right" amount of exercise is entirely relative and subjective, but in most cases, it's probably a lot less than you think. See the section "Keeping it simple: The secret to a good fitness program" for details.

Promoting beautiful movement

The third principle of Paleo fitness states that exercise should promote beautiful movement and stimulate a positive hormonal response. Just as trudging on the treadmill is equal to committing biomechanical treason so is crushing yourself day in and day out by lifting weights. One promotes a dysfunctional movement pattern (gait) and the other a negative long-term hormonal response (overtraining). But conventional fitness practices manage to overlook this detail, as big-box gyms pummel the masses with a less than choice exercise selection. Injury rates are high and retention low. Go figure.

With Paleo fitness, you marry beautiful movement with beautiful food, which results in a strong, beautiful body.

Keeping it simple: The secret to a good fitness program

Any exercise (and nutrition) program will improve in direct proportion to the number of things that you can keep out of it that don't need to be there. In other words, the secret to a good exercise program is to strip it down to the fewest possible parts — the fundamentals — and leave it at that. Paleo fitness is all about simplicity.

The fundamentals of Paleo are simple and proven effective. All you have to do is follow a simple diet of meats, eggs, fish, veggies, nuts, seeds, and *some* fruit. Then move often and move beautifully, lift heavy every couple of days, and occasionally run for your life (just not on a treadmill).

The secret is to practice strength selectively. We estimate that about 20 tried-and-true exercises — which probably amounts to less than 5 percent of all the exercises out there — are guaranteed to get you 95 percent of all the results you could ever want.

And just as you carefully choose how to move, be selective in what you eat, too. You need to eat less — not necessarily fewer calories but less variety and less frequently. Eat the same Paleo foods often, but eat them infrequently.

When it comes to fitness, we agree with the saying "all change is decay." Keep it simple with the fundamentals, and you'll do all right.

Getting Results: The Paleo Payoff

Although we'd love to say that following the Paleo fitness program is easy, successful lifestyle changes seldom come without their trials and tribulations. However, we promise that this book, and the workouts contained herein, will return to you exactly what you put in. The returns are 1:1, precisely. And that's the best you'll find anywhere.

Paleo fitness is grounded in good science, and good science produces predictable and repeatable results — that is, what can happen to one, can happen to all. In this section, we review some of those expectations — and results.

With Paleo fitness, you get out of it exactly what you put in. We give you everything you need to succeed, but ultimately, your success depends on your ability to take action.

Seeing is believing: Visual results

Most people want results and want them now. But nothing worthwhile ever comes fast and easy. The problem here is improperly set expectations. People are promised "fast and easy," but when they don't get it, they quit. This isn't what Paleo fitness is about. We're not selling any delusions here, only proven and sustainable methods — all of which require a considerable amount of effort on your part.

Now to address the most pressing question about any fitness program, the answer is, yes, you absolutely will lose weight with Paleo fitness. And the process won't be long, tedious, or painful, either. In fact, with the Paleo workouts in this book, six-pack abs are not only easily obtainable but almost inevitable. This result is merely a consequence of moving you into your ideal body fat range, which for men is between 8 to 12 percent and for women, 16 to 22 percent. (If you're unsure of your body fat percentage and want to get the most accurate reading, we recommend seeking out a facility that has a BOD POD body fat measuring device. Otherwise, you can simply hire a trainer who knows how to conduct a 7-point caliper test.) Then all you have to do is stick to the program.

Paleo fitness helps build your strength, too — not bulky strength but real-world functional strength. In other words, you'll gain the lean and wiry strength of a cave man, which is a good thing because life is easier when you're strong.

You may also expect noticeable changes in movement quality. Your everyday flexibility and mobility will improve when you begin to mobilize. Stiffness will turn to suppleness, and you'll no longer feel as wound up as a spring or as tight as a wheel clamp.

What's equally exciting is how you'll feel on the inside. With Paleo fitness, you'll notice stark differences in sleep quality, energy levels, and mental focus. Expect to beat that sluggish feeling once and for all — without the danger of harmful supplements or unnatural energy boosters.

Knowing what's going on behind the scenes: Other results

Equally important to looking your best is feeling your best. And we think you'll be delighted to experience all the benefits of Paleo fitness that extend far beyond the realm of "looking good naked."

For example, when you incorporate Paleo workouts into your life, you'll experience fewer illness and ailments. The Paleo diet has come to be known for its marvelous ability to boost immunity — and these effects are only greatly enhanced when you add Paleo fitness into the batter. And if you suffer from allergies, don't be surprised if they start to alleviate, too. Results such as these are typical.

To give you an idea, here's a brief list of what you can expect to improve through Paleo fitness:

- Hunger control
- Blood sugar regulation
- Improved joint and bone health
- Alleviated allergies and less sickness
- Increased energy levels and concentration
- Enhanced cellular function and physical performance

A Primal Primer: What You Need to Get Started

The cave man was a minimalist. He was a simple man and enjoyed simple things. His language displayed no fancy technique; in fact, he spoke in clicks, "tsk tsk" and "clop clop." It was horse talk mostly.

The cave man's diet was also quite unpretentious. He ate mostly tubers (yams, radishes, and rutabaga), fish, and game meat. No sugar, and very little, if any, grains or dairy.

When referring to the cave man, we think "hunter-gatherer," but it's probably more accurate to say "scavenger-gatherer," meaning he picked meat from carcasses and preyed upon easy prey — namely, the dead or pretty much dead. A bit crude, and perhaps a tad less dignified, but who are we to judge?

Interestingly, but not surprisingly, the cave man had a higher percentage of muscle than people do today, because of his intense and often heavy physical labors. The cave man would often walk, sprint, hang, hinge, squat, push, pull, throw, and carry. Because of this, the cave man was lean, strong, and durable — a product of hard living.

All of these things are lessons mostly on how to eat well and how to move beautifully. In the following sections, we outline what you need to get started on your Paleo fitness journey.

Going low-tech for high impact

We've searched long and hard, up and down, over the river and through the woods, but nothing we've ever come across on our quest for physical excellence has yet to impress us as the human body itself.

You can gain strength, power, and aesthetics — vastly superior to that of the average individual indentured at the big-box gym — quickly, safely, and inexpensively through a choice selection of primal bodyweight exercises. Paleo fitness demands that you unplug, disconnect, and go low-tech to reap high yield. In fact, the primal exercises requiring little to no equipment often produce the biggest results and need no warming up to.

For example, take the wonderful elasticity of the push-up: an exercise that can be tailored to any individual at any experience level. The beginner who lacks upper body strength may start by performing the push-up on an incline (against a wall), whereas the veteran may perpetually challenge and elevate his strength via the one-arm push-up or the one-arm one-leg push-up.

If there's a most important distinction on why Paleo fitness focuses heavily on bodyweight exercises, aside from their astounding cost-to-benefit ratio, then it's because they're both easily scalable and progressive:

- ✔ *Scaling* exercise is either toning it down or blaring it up. For example, the push-up is easily scaled in difficulty by increasing or decreasing the angle (elevating the hands or the feet), or by adding or subtracting limbs (two-arm push-up versus one-arm push-up), or most simply, by adding or subtracting repetitions.

- ✔ Providing a *progression,* on the other hand, is to provide a clear and logical path toward advancement or a higher skill. And to progress to the push-up — that is, to do a push-up properly — you need to start with the plank, similar to how you first learn to crawl before you walk.

In other words, progressions is learning how to do something, and scalability is making something doable.

Most conventional fitness practices offer scalability (making something easier or harder) but little in the ways of progressions (teaching how to do something properly). And that's a dangerous game to play. However, we offer both.

Choosing the kettlebell to enhance and extend

The kettlebell is a brutish but brilliant device. It's a hunk of iron with a handle slapped on it: ugly, heavy, superb.

When used properly, the kettlebell merely forms an extension of the body, and because you can swing it, throw it, carry it, press it, squat it, snatch it, jerk it, lunge it, and so on, it's the prime implement to mimic the rigors and heavy lifting of a primal lifestyle.

The kettlebell also fills in the few holes left behind by bodyweight training. To wit: The kettlebell is a tool that, when employed properly, will help you move powerfully, efficiently, and gracefully.

In addition to your own bodyweight, you can use any number of tools to mimic the labors of the cave man, but not all of them do the job quite as well as the kettlebell. In other words, for any given task, a plethora of tools may help you get the job done, but you need to choose the tool that gets the job done best, and that is the kettlebell.

Although you can do many of the workouts in this book with body weight alone, using a kettlebell enhances and extends your movement so you get better results, faster. And lucky for you, we show you just how to use the kettlebell and use it well to make the most of your Paleo fitness journey.

Getting rid of the "necessities"

Necessary for the participation in any given conventional fitness routine is a list of stuff that's always pretentious, expensive, and wrong. These are the "must gets," or what many may label as true necessities for fitness; they include fancy footwear, highfalutin apparel, exaggerated supplements, affected heart rate monitor — and so on and so on.

But if you want to work out and work out well, the truth is that all you need is a pulse. Everything else is either a bonus or a distraction.

The Paleo fitness aficionado is an ultra-light traveler, toting only the bare minimum necessities, and aims to mimic the cave man, who was, after all, a fitness vagabond (if there ever was such a thing). His gym was all of Earth. He cared nothing for dumbbells as he lifted stones, logs, and carcasses. He cared even less for treadmills as he sprinted regularly outdoors to hunt and to avoid being hunted. And besides, he'd have nowhere to plug one in.

So with Paleo fitness, our list of "must gets" is mostly short and, aside from a set of kettlebells (see previous section), already complete. However, we provide you with a list of "must get rid-ofs" in the following sections.

Ditch the shoes

By now, you may have begun to notice a trend in the Paleo community that began picking up steam a few years back with the release of a book called *Born to Run* (Vintage), where author Christopher McDougall makes a sound enough argument for barefoot running. Now, we're not for long, trudging runs. We don't think long runs are all that good for you, and we have evidence to support this theory (which we roll out in Chapter 9). Nevertheless, the occasional jog that's both light and bouncy is a marvelous way to keep on the move. And save for a few unusual circumstances, it's best performed barefoot.

So are we saying that you should dismiss shoes from your feet and embrace an entirely barefoot lifestyle? The answer is no. That'd be silly. Shoes were invented for a reason, such as to avoid stepping on glass, nails, and jagged rocks, so they still serve a purpose.

If you've been in shoes all your life, ease your way into barefoot running and lifting. To avoid injury, you must give your feet, ankles, and calves ample time to adapt. Don't do too much too soon.

When it comes to Paleo fitness, barefoot is the way to go for these reasons:

- ✔ **Greater support/stability:** Exercising and lifting weights in shoes, particularly shoes with a lot of cushion or heel, is almost like lifting on a mattress. It's unstable. And when it comes to lifting heavy things, you want the most stable base of support you can get. When you ditch the shoes and go barefoot, you can root yourselves to the ground and secure a more stable position.

- ✔ **Better lifting form:** Few shoes are designed with heavy front squats or dead lifts in mind, so few shoes promote proper lifting mechanics. For example, a shoe with a lot of heel naturally edges the weight forward — toward the front of the foot — which is precisely where you don't want it to be when squatting, lunging, dead lifting, and so on, because it translates to greater stress on the knees and the low back. Consequently, when you ditch the shoes, you may shift your weight back toward your heels and lift more from your hips and less from your knees or back.

✔ **Stronger feet, ankles, and calves:** Shoes put the muscles of the feet, ankles, and calves out of work, either in part or in whole. In turn, they grow weak and dysfunctional, which puts you at a higher risk for injury. Without shoes, the artificial support is gone and your lowermost extremities must go back to work, so they grow stronger, and you're less likely to fall into injury.

✔ **Increased proprioception/bodily awareness:** The bottoms of your feet have sensors that pick up and transmit valuable information to your brain about your position and orientation in space — called *proprioception*. Shoes often distort or misinterpret these signals, and subsequently, the quality of your movement suffers.

The less shoe, the better, we say. But if for whatever reason you can't go strictly barefoot, then opt for minimalist footwear, such as Vibram Five Fingers, New Balance Minimus, or if you're feeling bold, a pair of flip flops.

Cancel the gym membership

Do you need a gym membership to implement a Paleo fitness program? Not at all. Will it help? It can't hurt. If nothing else, it can provide equipment such as kettlebells, dumbbells, and barbells, for your Paleo fitness journey. Just be sure to steer clear of the equipment you don't need, like the treadmills, ellipticals, and exercise machines.

We're quite keen on working out outdoors, and there's certainly something to be said about training *alfresco*. It's primal. It feels good. And you get your daily dose of sunlight. Whether you choose to cancel your gym membership is entirely up to you, but we encourage you to break your Paleo fitness routine out into the sunlight every now and then.

Dismiss preconceived notions

One last thing to purge before you begin your Paleo fitness journey is any and all preconceived notions that you have about fitness and health. You'll soon find that Paleo fitness is marked by minimalism, which is precisely what makes it such a good fitness program.

In fact, Paleo fitness has in it all that you look for in a significant other but rarely find. It's uncluttered and unfussy. It never tires you unfairly. And when you need some time off, it doesn't make you feel guilty about it.

Chapter 2

The Things You Ought to Do: Proper Cave Man Etiquette

In This Chapter

▶ Realizing the importance of strength training

▶ Moving and breathing like you were designed to do

▶ Identifying what compels you to get fit and healthy

▶ Discovering the most effective and efficient exercise practices

▶ Understanding the power of fasting and the Paleo diet

*B*efore you get into the primal exercise routines and get to work in Parts II and III, we provide a few techniques in this chapter that will guarantee your success and, more importantly, your safety.

In Chapter 1, we talk about Paleo principles and values. In brief, we talk about *Paleo strategy* —the things you need to do to achieve vibrant health, a sexier physique, and peak performance. Here, we talk about *Paleo tactics* — the things you should do specifically. These tactics are the finer details. Some may even go so far as to call them minor details. But keep these words in mind: Big doors swing on little hinges. Often, the littlest tweaks produce the largest results.

In this chapter, we present nine simple techniques that everyone should do on a regular basis. For this set of guidelines, we've reverse-engineered the lifestyle of the cave man.

All the techniques in this chapter are immediately applicable, and the quicker you put them into practice, the quicker you'll start dropping weight and building muscle, the quicker you'll start feeling vibrant and vivacious, and the quicker you can close this book! We'll even go so far as to say that anyone who practices these simple techniques 90 percent of the time will see 99 percent of his remediable health issues rapidly remedied.

Cultivate Strength

This chapter was a difficult one for us to write, mostly because we couldn't decide on the proper order of the things you ought to do. And even though we believe that the first thing is just as important as the last, there's always an implication — albeit a small one — that what comes first is more significant. And so, recognizing this, we put strength first. Just to play it safe. Indeed, many valuable attributes exist, from agility and balance to anaerobic/aerobic capacity, flexibility, mobility, but before anything else, you ought to cultivate strength.

In this section, we explain what it means to cultivate strength by first defining what strength is and then showing you how strength helps you build a strong foundation for the other things you ought to do.

Knowing what strength really is

Throughout our pursuits, we've come across many workable but somewhat lacking definitions for strength. For example, a haughty and somewhat respectable lifter once said that true strength is a 500-pound dead lift, a 400-pound squat, and a 300-pound bench press. On the other end of the spectrum, poet Judith Viorst says that strength is the ability to break a chocolate bar into four pieces with your bare hands.

Finally, one definition in particular has always struck us as both beautiful and correct and is stated simply as this: Strength is the ability to overcome resistance.

Resistance comes in many forms — mental, physical, internal, external — it's any force in opposition of what you're trying to do. And the only way to gain strength is to work against resistance.

For example, the push-up provides resistance of your own body weight. But by working against this resistance, you develop upper body strength.

Getting stronger to fix just about everything

We subscribe to the general theory that being strong fixes just about everything, insofar that we've been offering one simple, sweeping, and effective antidote to the general ailments of the masses: Get strong(er).

Here are just a few benefits of primal strength training:

- ✔ Decreased fat mass
- ✔ Improved focus/concentration
- ✔ Improved glucose tolerance (decreased risk of diabetes)
- ✔ Improved heart health
- ✔ Improved sleep quality
- ✔ Increased lean body mass
- ✔ Increased stamina
- ✔ Reduced risk of injury
- ✔ Stress relief
- ✔ Stronger bones (decreased risk of osteoporosis)

General bodily weakness inhibits everything, whereas the stronger you are (the more force you can produce), the easier everything else becomes. In other words, as you increase your strength capacity, you increase all capacities, including but not limited to the following:

- ✔ Muscular endurance — the ability to exert force over a prolonged period of time
- ✔ Cardiovascular endurance — the ability to sustain strenuous cardiovascular efforts for a prolonged period of time
- ✔ Power — how much force you can produce in a given amount of time
- ✔ Coordination — how well everything in your body plays together

So strength is the foundation on which everything else is built, and it's generally useless to train anything else without training strength first. Consider this: Will the firefighter who trains for strength or the firefighter who trains for endurance be able to perform his tasks with greater efficiency? The answer is the one who trains for strength because if the one who trains for endurance has no strength base — that is, if he's unable to lift the equipment or unable to drag an unresponsive person — then his general endurance is unusable. His endurance training has been for not.

Endurance is only possible to the extent that you're stronger than the task at hand, meaning that lifting and carrying a 150-pound body will be an easy act of endurance for the person who can lift 300 pounds but an impossible task for the person who can lift only 75 pounds. To say it another way, the person who can lift 300 pounds even once will have no trouble lifting 100 pounds many times, but the person who can lift 100 pounds many times may not be able to lift 300 pounds even once. To understand this is to know that increasing strength increases endurance but not the other way around.

Endurance is simply a byproduct of strength. If you want to improve your endurance, get stronger!

Developing strength as a skill

The cave man was strong because strength was requisite for survival. But today, this whole business of strength often presents a dilemma. People think that strength is an attribute of the genetically gifted and that if they picked the wrong parents, they're out of luck.

Strength isn't hereditary; it's a skill, in the same vein that skiing, typing, or learning a new language are all skills. A skill is a habit of operation, something you acquire through observation and experience. You learn the rules, and then you operate according to the rules until you form a habit. In other words, you learn by doing.

So if you lack strength, it's not because you chose the wrong parents but because you chose the wrong habits. Therefore, if you're weak, you either aren't practicing effective habits or you're practicing ineffective habits.

Skills range in complexity. For example, learning a new language or how to play the piano are complex skills that take years to develop (at least to a level of significant proficiency). Strength, however, is a simple skill — one that anyone at any age can acquire rapidly. So just as a pianist acquires the skill of musicianship through diligent practice, you acquire strength in the same way. But instead of running scales, you lift weights.

Furthermore, skills also range in necessity. If you're unable to moonwalk, you need not offer any apologies. That's a hard skill to master and is relatively useless. Strength, however, is essential, and there's no excuse for not cultivating that skill. For strength — true strength — you need to follow only two simple rules:

- **Practice often.** We don't know anyone who has ever acquired a skill without practice. Strength is no exception. If you want to get strong at pull-ups, practice pull-ups. If you want to get strong at squats, practice squats.

- **Lift heavy some of the time.** We can't say this more plainly. If you want to get strong — really strong, that is — then you have to push your limits every so often. Not every day, but every couple of days you want to lift heavy and push yourself.

Realizing there's more to fitness than strength

Lifting heavy is all very well and primal. And torn sinew, from time to time, just *feels* good. But we must warn you that strength can be a little addicting. And as you probably know, too much of any one good thing can quickly turn it bad.

Although we tell you to train strength first, you don't want to do so exclusively or excessively. Strength is the capacity that lifts all other capacities, but it doesn't necessarily fill them. As your strength increases, so does the potential for endurance, flexibility, conditioning, and so on.

Prioritize strength, but don't neglect everything else. We've seen many strong athletes trample because they failed to give heed to their heart, and we've seen many strong lifters get injured because they paid no mind to the quality of their movement. Chasing strength and strength alone is a foolish and down-right dangerous crusade.

So after this puzzling realization, you may be wondering "what else are we to do?" This fundamental question deserves a fundamental answer. And that answer, of course, is everything else, covered conveniently in the rest of this chapter.

Move Every Day

Life is movement. And the opposite of movement is motionlessness, which you could say is an apt definition of death. The cave man was constantly on the move in one way or another so he suffered few of the problems that people do today, problems brought about largely from a lack of quality movement.

As people age and take on more responsibilities, they tend to slip into stillness. They sit too much, and they get rigid. They fail to move, and so they start to creak like the tin man.

This pattern is unfortunate but highly preventable and, if it has already set in, easily remediable. A life rich in movement wards off the deleterious effects of aging. It keeps the cells fresh, the muscles toughened, and the joints well oiled. And if life is movement, then surely movement stimulates life — it rejuvenates muscle tissue, upsurges joint nutrition, and even spurs the growth of new brain cells.

When we say you need to move every day, we don't mean that you have to work out with great intensity every day; just move. When you plan how to move every day, keep it easy, but do it often. We offer up our favorite recommendations and show you how to do them in Chapter 3.

There's no such thing as a wrong movement. You can suffer only from a lack of movement.

For now, a few basic human movement patterns every day will suffice. Explore new positions, postures, and patterns, like the following:

✔ Bend	✔ March
✔ Carry	✔ Pull
✔ Crawl	✔ Push
✔ Flex	✔ Roll
✔ Hang	✔ Rotate
✔ Hinge	✔ Squat
✔ Jump	✔ Throw
✔ Lunge	✔ Twist

Don't confuse movement with exercise. Although exercise includes movement, the means and the ends aren't the same. Exercise induces stress and is often intense, such as five sets of five heavy reps on the back squat. Movement promotes rejuvenation and is usually lighthearted and playful, such as crawling around on the ground with a newborn.

Breathe Every Day

Through simple deductive reasoning — that is, you're alive, therefore, you're breathing — we can deduce that you've met the simple act of breathing with a considerable amount of success. However, breathing is too complex and influential a task to be graded like finger painting or Lego blocks. And the type of breathing we're talking about isn't the involuntary act of breathing but the conscious type. We explore the types of breathing and how they affect your health in the following sections.

Breathing affects everything

Human respiration — the seemingly simple act of breathing — is perhaps the most powerful regulatory agency in the body. The rate and depth of your breath has the power to arouse and depress the senses, and it has long been known that you can affect your mood simply and rapidly by changing your breathing.

Breathing affects everything from your mood to the quality of your sleep. Don't discount the benefits of taking a few minutes every day to practice deep, purposeful breathing.

Overbreathing — often referred to as *hyperventilation* — is where your breath is laborious and excessive. If you've ever had a panic attack, you've experienced hyperventilation and know it's frightening. Hyperventilating is paralyzing and sorely limits your ability to perform under stress.

Mostly, people just breathe too often. If you're taking more than 12 breaths a minute, you're overbreathing. Overbreathing, or hyperventilation, arouses anxiety (sometimes to the point of inducing panic), impairs cognition (sometimes to the point of memory loss), and promotes restlessness (sometimes to the point of insomnia).

Here are a few consequences of overbreathing:

- Anxiety
- Chronic fatigue
- Headaches
- Restlessness
- Stress

Abnormal breathing patterns, such as overbreathing, have been linked to a plethora of illnesses, from the vexatious (gastritis) to the deadly (heart disease).

Breathing the way you were meant to breathe

When we say breathe every day, we mean that you should *breathe consciously* every day — that is, you should practice slow, rhythmic, diaphragmatic breathing. Babies breathe this way, long and deep into the belly.

Conscious breathing is more about the exhalation than it is the inhalation. To practice conscious breathing, you breathe in for a count of four and breathe out for a count of eight. If you take the time to do this slow breathing every day, as often as possible, your efforts will be well rewarded. When you control your breath, you control your composure, your deliberation, and, to a certain degree, your aging.

Take five minutes now to try the following breathing exercise, known as *crocodile breathing:*

1. **Lie flat on your belly and rest your forehead on your hands.**

2. **Slowly draw in a breath as deep into your belly as possible for four counts.**

   Your belly should push out into the ground, and your sides should also have some outward visible movement. Your shoulders and chest, however, shouldn't rise.

3. **Hold the breathe for a count of one, and then slowly exhale for a count of eight.**

Know What Compels You

People work out for two reasons: to move toward something, such as a heavier dead lift or a more chiseled midsection, and/or to move away from something, such as stiffness or poor self-esteem.

In the following sections, we show you how to identify what compels you to work out and how to set goals for fitness that you can stick to.

Identifying your primal motivators

Some people choose to work out because they want to be something they're not, and some people choose to work out because they want to stop being something they are. Some people work out for vanity — they want to whittle their waistline, tighten their butts, or carve out their abs to look like the sinewy superstar cover model — and there's nothing wrong with that. And then some people work out for glory — they want to be an elite athlete, they want to crush the competition, and they want to do so mercilessly in front of thousands of raving fans — and there's nothing wrong with that, either.

These are just common examples of working out to move toward something. People want to get to somewhere new, and they want to be someone new. The promise of pleasure compels them. And there's certainly nothing wrong with that.

The other reason is slightly less sexy but slightly more common. It's when people work out because they feel like they have to or because the doctor said if they don't, they'll have a heart attack and die. It's when they look into the mirror and see that their arms are soft and doughy, like a pair of breadsticks, and that their stomach has grown outward — in a geometrical fashion — like The Blob. It's typically a revolting reality, and people will suddenly do anything to move away from such a poor self-image.

People reach a point, often a very painful point, where they're so disgusted and fed up with themselves that they just can't take it any longer. Something needs to be done. They don't necessarily care where they go, as long as they get away from where they're at right now. Most people have been there at one time or another.

Whatever the reason may be, you need to know why you're working out, and you need to remind yourself of that reason daily — because that's what compels you.

Everyone seeks fitness either to avoid pain or to gain pleasure (sometimes both). Identifying and understanding what compels you and them reminding yourself daily will help you stick to the program.

Setting goals that stick

When it comes to setting goals, of any sort, it's best to aim high — higher even than you suspect you may be able to reach — and in many circumstances, it's best to forgo what's easily obtainable for something that's really going to challenge you. Even if you fail, chances are that you'll still land a lot higher than you would otherwise. Additionally, setting goals that are a bit lofty is enthralling. And goals that are enthralling tend to have a higher stick rate.

Set yourself a goal that excites you, regardless of how crazy it sounds. Boring goals rarely stick, because they're, well, boring! Get creative. Get a little rambunctious, even. And go for what you truly want.

Although losing two pounds may be a goal of yours, it's hard to get very excited about meeting that goal. So set a goal for yourself that's a bit more imaginative and, dare we say, loftier. For example, imagine that the editors of some glamorous publication want to feature you on the cover as the "best body of the year." All you have to do is get ready for the shoot. Now doesn't that sounds like something worth working toward?

On the other hand, you want to be sure to set goals that are humanly possible and that you're actually able to achieve in the amount of time you've given yourself to achieve them. There's a difference between aiming high and being completely unrealistic.

To this end, you should set *S.M.A.R.T.* goals that meet the following criteria:

- ✔ **Specific:** For example, "I want to lose weight" isn't a specific goal, but "I want to lose five pounds" is. Do your best to make your goals as specific as possible.

- ✔ **Measurable:** You should be able to measure your progress along the way. If you can't, then how will you ever know whether you're making any progress? Luckily, most fitness-related goals are measurable. Losing body fat is measurable (via body fat analysis) and so is gaining strength (via strength testing).

- ✔ **Attainable:** Although you want to set lofty goals, you don't want to set unrealistic goals. If you set goals that are entirely out of your current reach, you're only setting yourself up for failure and disappointment. You need to set goals that challenge you but that you can achieve so you get a feeling of accomplishment, which will motivate you to reach other goals.

- ✔ **Relevant:** For our purposes here, all your goals should be fitness-related. Although being more fit and healthy may very well make you more productive at work, setting the goal of getting that promotion you've really wanted in three months is hardly relevant here.

- ✔ **Time-bound:** There's a saying that "a goal without a deadline is simply a dream." We agree. Without a clear-cut deadline, you have no reason not to procrastinate. So give yourself a deadline, one that's realistic but also pressing enough to give yourself the impetus you need to get to work!

Train the Primal Patterns Primarily

Up to a point, we support the proposition that you can get 95 percent of all the strength and fitness you'll ever need from 5 percent of all the exercises you've ever heard of and subtle variations therein. In other words, a handful of battlefield-tested exercises offer tremendous utility — far above and beyond that of most other exercises.

This proposition is a spin on the *Pareto principal,* or what's more commonly referred to as the *80/20 rule.* Simply put, the 80/20 rule states that 80 percent of all effects come from 20 percent of the causes. Commonly, a pea garden illustrates this phenomenon, demonstrating that 80 percent of the peas grown in any one garden are often the result of only 20 percent of the pea pods.

The 80/20 rule can and has been applied to increase the efficiency of tasks in multiple domains. In business, it commonly reveals that 20 percent of customers contribute 80 percent of the income.

And as you may suspect, it can even be applied to fitness, although we tend to think the ratio is probably a bit more skewed — more like 95 percent of all the results you could ever want come from 5 percent of all the possible things that you could ever do. And this 5 percent consists of the fundamental primal human movements, of which there are roughly six:

- Pushing
- Pulling
- Hinging
- Squatting
- Carrying
- Walking and sprinting (gait)

We review these movements in the following sections.

Pushing

A *push* isn't an exercise per se but rather a category of movement. It includes the push-up (see Figure 2-1), the military press, and the bench press, all of which are big pushes. And if we were forced to rank them, we'd rank them just in that order: best, better, and still great.

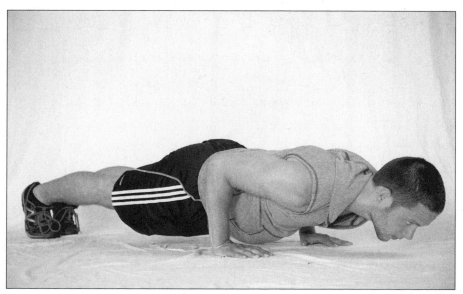

Figure 2-1: The push-up is the king of pushes.

Photo courtesy of Rebekah Ulmer

Within each category of human movement, you want to do the movements that offer the highest return on investment. The push does that. And the push-up in particular is perhaps the perfect primal exercise, working trunk stability and upper-body pushing strength. This classic gym class exercise strengthens the chest, shoulders, triceps, and abs.

Pulling

Now when we talk about pulling, surely we mean the pull-up (see Figure 2-2) because we've found nothing finer for a strong and muscular back.

Don't fret if you're unable to perform even one rep of the pull-up, and certainly don't listen to the bunkum recently churned out claiming that "females can't do pull-ups." Females most certainly *can* and most certainly *should* do pull-ups. Anyone who says otherwise has never had enough strength — or brains — to know better. We've trained many females from zero to five pull-ups within two months' time. That's more than most males can do, and we can get you there, too.

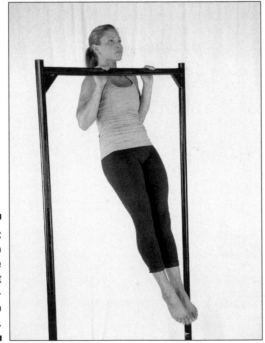

Figure 2-2:
The pull-up
is the
perfect
primal com-
plement to
the push-up.

Photo courtesy of Rebekah Ulmer

Hinging

Hinging — a movement horribly underpracticed — is a tremendously useful pattern, and throughout this book, we practice it diligently with what is perhaps the most marvelous fat-chopping device ever seen: the kettlebell swing. Hinging forges an iron posterior and is, or at least should be, the default movement pattern for picking stuff up off the ground.

As an athlete, you can produce a tremendous amount of force from a hinge — think of a lineman before the snap, a sprinter before the gun, or a broad jumper before the leap; these actions are all strong and all come out of a hinged position. Figure 2-3 shows the dead lift, which is perhaps the most common hinging pattern of all. The dead lift strengthens the hips and the back. When performing the dead lift, be sure to keep the back flat and the hips below the shoulders but above the knees. (See Chapter 5 for full instructions on this movement.)

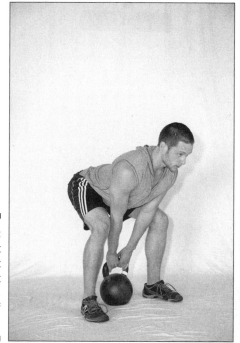

Figure 2-3:
The dead lift is the best movement for picking stuff up off the ground.

Photo courtesy of Rebekah Ulmer

Squatting

In the category of the squat, we venture the recommendations of the goblet squat, the pistol squat, and the front squat — all of which we cover in great depth in Chapter 5. The squat is an essential human movement pattern. It keeps the hips supple and the knees strong. It's also a natural rest position, meaning that you should be able to get down into a squat and sit there comfortably for extended periods of time.

Figure 2-4 shows the primal or bodyweight squat. If you have the mobility, it should feel almost effortless to sit in the bottom position of this squat. You want to try to accumulate as much time as you can in the bottom of a squat position throughout the day. Doing so will work wonders for your hips, knees, and back.

Figure 2-4:
The primal squat, or the bodyweight squat, should serve as a natural rest position.

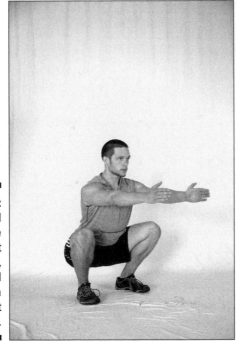

Photo courtesy of Rebekah Ulmer

Carrying

We can't think of a single movement pattern more primal — or more useful — than the basic carrying of heavy objects. You do it every day, so it's quite important, we think.

Carrying, as strength coach Dan John would say, "fills in the gaps." It's something that everyone should do, but most people don't. Carrying helps reinforce proper posture (which is often neglected) and strengthens the grip (finger and forearm strength is also paid very little attention). Throughout the book, we employ the waiter's carry, the farmer's carry (see Figure 2-5), and the Turkish get-up to "fill in the gaps."

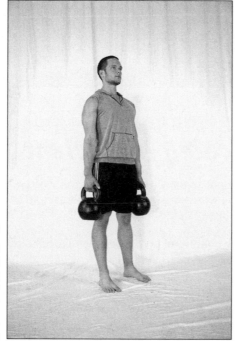

Figure 2-5:
Carries
truly earn
the title of
"functional"
exercise.

Photo courtesy of Rebekah Ulmer

Walking and sprinting

Gait, or the manner of moving on foot, includes walking and sprinting (see Figure 2-6). Jogging, especially for long distances, is a dreadful undertaking, and we don't recommend it. Instead, you should steep yourself primarily in the two ends of the force-velocity spectrum. You should move slowly very often and move very fast occasionally. There's little benefit to playing around in the middle (jogging).

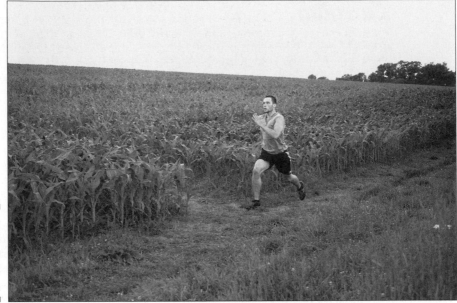

Photo courtesy of Rebekah Ulmer

Figure 2-6: If you need to move quickly, sprint.

Keep Your Conditioning Inefficient

As with anything else, a heap of semantics surrounds the word *conditioning*. People argue that conditioning means a great many things, and they're right. Conditioning is a word with many definitions.

But for our purposes, we link conditioning to anything related to the strengthening of the heart muscle, and more thrillingly, fat loss. We explain in detail what conditioning is and how you should approach it in the following sections.

Conditioning for strength or fat loss

Strength is efficiency. It's a finely tuned nervous system, if you will. For example, a more efficient person can produce more force with the same amount of muscle than a less-efficient person; in other words, he uses his brawny resources more resourcefully.

The fewer moving parts, the more efficient a machine becomes. Although you're not a machine, this analogy still serves a useful purpose. Your movement, from the standpoint of strength, shouldn't consume any more than the bare minimum effort required. This, of course, takes practice.

But, for conditioning — moreover, fat loss — you don't want to strive for efficiency. Quite the opposite really. Because the more efficient you become, the less energy you expend, and the more difficult it is to drop pounds, which is another reason long, trudging runs are comparatively futile for fat loss. They may produce measly returns upfront, but those returns are quickly and severely diminished when you become an efficient jogger. And even if you're not an efficient jogger yet, jogging by itself is a more efficient means of travel than, say, sprinting is — you expend considerably more energy sprinting 50 yards than you do jogging that same distance.

So if you want to fight fat effectively, you need to fight it with inefficiency. You need to select movements and exercise protocols that are wasteful in terms of energy expenditure, such as sprinting and various metabolic conditioning routines.

Comparing efficiency and effectiveness

Naturally, to do something efficiently is to do something economically. Efficiency is easily measured by the ratio of input to output (how much you get for what you give). In the example of jogging versus sprinting, jogging is more efficient because you give less (energy) to get the same result (distance traveled).

Efficiency is also easily measured qualitatively by your perceived level of exertion. To wit: The more challenging or difficult an exercise or exercise regimen feels, the less efficient it probably is.

Effectiveness, on the other hand, has little to do with economy but more to do with ability — that is, the ability to produce a desired result. Effectiveness, unlike efficiency, isn't so easily quantified. In other words, effectiveness is *doing the right things,* whereas efficiency is *doing things right.* A chief distinction between the two is that just because something is efficient doesn't mean it's effective (and vice versa).

One example is step aerobics; another is Zumba. These exercises are efficient — as made clear by the relatively low level of exertion — but relatively useless weaponry for the battle against body fat.

Low-intensity aerobics, such as walking or hiking, are tremendously beneficial for overall health, and you should do them often. By themselves, however, they are ineffective for rapid changes in body composition.

So if your aim is to combat fat, effectively and unapologetically, then you need to downgrade to a more primitive arsenal. Do it in the way of the cave man, and really exert yourself. Sprint hard, lift heavy, and play often.

Do the Least You Have to Do

The idea that a perpetually enlarging dose of exercise — that is, spending a lot of time in the gym — will continue to improve the body's function and appearance indefinitely is as unsound and nearly as dangerous as the notion that the complexion and health of the skin will improve in direct ratio to the number of hours spent basking in the sun. Exercise is to be practiced judiciously. You want to do just enough to get the job done and not a smidgeon more.

Too much exercise can lead to a chronic state of stress known as overtraining. Here are some of the symptoms to look out for:

- Anxiety
- Depression
- Increased/abnormal heart rate
- Insomnia
- Low energy/chronic fatigue
- Low libido
- Memory problems
- Poor concentration
- Weight gain

The chief aim of exercise is to impose a demand on the bodily systems — to inject stress and subsequently force an adaptation. The body requires time to recover from the stress, and to adapt, you must rest.

When you inject more stress than you can accommodate, recovery is inhibited and you, at best, decelerate your progress and, at worst, die. Indeed, the latter is quite rare, but still, it can happen.

Intense exercise is a potent drug; a little does a lot of good, but a lot does very little good. In other words, if what you're doing is effective, the marginal returns are severely diminished after you've run the minimum dose. The minimum dose, or the *minimum effective dose* (MED) as Tim Ferriss refers to in his book *The 4-Hour Body* (Ebury), is "the smallest dose that will produce a desired outcome." Anything beyond the MED is simply wasteful. For example, if it takes only x number of reps to elicit the response you want, then don't do $x + 1$.

So how much is enough? The answer depends on what you want. But in any circumstance, it's probably less than you think.

Fast . . . Sometimes

The notion that you need to eat every couple of hours or so is one of the more fatuous delusions of conventional wisdom. We've tried — really, really hard — but failed to find anything supporting this idea that can even remotely be described as sound scientific evidence.

The frequent feeding frenzy was popularized by bodybuilders sometime in the 1980s, when it was proper etiquette to work two twice-baked potatoes, 12 cheesy eggs, and a side of woolly mammoth into your system at any and all junctures. How this madness ever became convention — or widely accepted as "the healthy thing to do" — or how people came to believe that it "speeds up your metabolism" is beyond us. Any study we've seen attempting to substantiate these claims rings up as "inconclusive," is as poorly planned, calculated, and executed as a family vacation, or proves the contrary.

And interestingly enough, a lot of evidence supports the contrary — that is, the benefits of fasting and infrequent feeding. By the way, *fasting* is any lengthy abstinence from food. It's not eating for a while — anywhere from 16 to 24 hours. *Infrequent feeding* is equally self-descriptive: Eat less often throughout the day, about two to three meals a day. (Four to six meals a day is considered *frequent feeding*.)

The following sections show you exactly why sometimes fasting is beneficial.

Fasting helps you lose weight (and keep it off)

Fasting is a safe, effective, and sustainable means for fat loss. Not eating will help you shed pounds. The daft notion of "starvation mode" has been carried out to truly preposterous lengths. True starvation mode — or true *adaptive thermogenesis,* to be more precise — is a long-term adaptation to severe caloric restriction. An occasional break from eating, even a break of up to 24 hours, won't throw you into starvation mode; it won't "slow down your metabolism," and it won't make you gain weight.

To maintain order, all nature ebbs and flows: the tides, the moons, the seasons, and even the economy. In nature, cyclicality is normal, whereas fixity is really quite unnatural. You also need an ebb and flow between hunger and satiety to keep optimum health. But conventional wisdom fears hunger like a hobgoblin. "Don't ever get hungry again," they say. "Keep the belly full," they say. Hunger is primal. Hunger is the hunt. It's motivation, activity to energy outflow. Get hungry, we say!

Don't duck, dodge, or sidestep fasting. Embrace it! Yes, fasting will help you cut pounds, but there's more to it than that: Fasting has demonstrated to specifically increase *lipolysis,* or fat burning. Losing weight is all well and good, but losing fat specifically is all the better.

Furthermore, fasting has also been proven effective to prevent *re-esterification* — taking fat back in after you've kicked it out. Losing fat is all well and good, but keeping it off is all the better.

Fasting keeps you young

If fasting hasn't snagged your interest yet, here's another benefit: Fasting promotes longevity and keeps the mind biologically young. Eating accelerates the aging process — that is, it speeds up the rate things start to sour biologically. So, then, not eating may slow the aging process.

It was once believed that overall calorie restriction prolonged life, but now feeding frequency plays an equal, if not more influential, role in the mystery of aging — because caloric restriction and fasting have both been shown to promote successful brain aging. Successful aging is aging free of neurological disease, as far as practicable, that is.

Now it may be somewhat premature to cast blame, but evidence suggests that unchecked insulin levels (*insulin* is a hormone secreted by the pancreas that regulates blood sugar and the primary nutrient transport hormone) may be mostly to blame for quickening the progression toward death and neurological disease. For example, certain scientific circles now think that Alzheimer's may actually be a form of diabetes — some have even gone so far as to call Alzheimer's Type 3 diabetes. What they're saying is that Alzheimer's is brought about by a lack of insulin receptors or poor sensitivity of insulin receptors in the brain. In short, Alzheimer's may in fact be a form of insulin resistance in the brain — or to be more direct, diabetes of the brain.

What does this have to do with fasting? Fasting improves insulin sensitivity. So the more you eat, the more insulin you secrete, and the less sensitive you become to it. You then have to secrete more insulin to get the job done. We refer to this cycle as the perpetual cycle of doom.

The only known way to break this cycle is to reverse it — that is, to eat less frequently and, therefore, secrete less insulin. Ultimately, the less insulin you secrete, the better off you are altogether.

Another reason infrequent feeding may promote longevity is because fasting has been shown to increase natural growth hormone, which provides the following benefits:

- ✔ More lean body mass
- ✔ Less fat mass (boosts metabolism by about 15 percent)
- ✔ Reduces stress and anxiety
- ✔ Improves concentration
- ✔ Enhances recovery from exercise
- ✔ Antiaging effects

Growth hormone makes for good health, plain and simple. And fasting increases both growth hormone pulse and frequency. This means you get more growth hormone more often.

Eat Like a Cave Man

The Paleo diet has caused quite a ruckus lately. But the benefits are now common knowledge — even the most obstinate of physicians and college professors can't help but acknowledge them.

Here are just a few of the benefits of the Paleo diet:

- ✔ Burns off body fat
- ✔ Clears skin
- ✔ Improves sleep
- ✔ Reduces allergies
- ✔ Stabilizes blood sugar

The rest of this section lays out the Paleo eating plan and shows you how to incorporate it into your life.

Eating the way you were designed to eat

The Paleo diet, also known as the cave man diet, is a way of eating that resembles the diet of our Paleolithic ancestors. It's a reversion to how people used to eat before the emergence of agriculture or the dawn of the Industrial Revolution. Really, it's how people were designed to eat.

The Paleo diet was first popularized as far back as the 1970s, but it really broke out into the mainstream to the sweet tune of Dr. Lorain Cordain's book *The Paleo Diet* (Houghton Mifflin), first published a few years back.

Since then, the Paleo diet has become nothing short of a welcome and timely phenomenon and has helped thousands upon thousands of people all around the world rejuvenate their bodies cell by cell. It also works quite marvelously for fat loss and muscle.

Eating Paleo means eating in accordance to your genetic blueprint. This diet isn't based on deprivation. The Paleo diet is about promoting a healthy gut and a healthy hormonal balance through the choicest selection of foods. The rules are few and simple:

- **Eat mostly meats, fish, and eggs.** Choose meats, such as beef and lamb; seafood, such as salmon, tuna, and sardines; poultry, such as chicken, turkey, and duck; and even organ meats. Organic meats are the best choice.

- **Eat a plethora of nutrient-rich vegetables.** Naturally, you should aim to eat the most nutrient-dense and lowest sugar vegetables possible, including spinach, kale, seaweeds, and most roots, shoots, and tubers.

- **Get plenty of healthy fats.** Get your healthy fats mostly from meats, nuts, seeds, and Paleo-approved oils. Coconut oil is one of the choicest cooking oils, and extra-virgin olive oil is a great oil to dress your salads with. Macadamia nuts, hazelnuts, and Brazil nuts are all great sources for healthy fats.

- **Eliminate all grains, dairy, and legumes.** Grains, dairy, and legumes all promote inflammation to various degrees. Chronic inflammation is a serious health matter leading to an almost limitless number of malaises and is often brought about from disagreeable food choices. Really, people were never designed to eat these foods, nor did they before the agriculture came about some 10,000 years ago. Either way, grains, dairy, or legumes don't contain any nutrients that you can't find elsewhere for fewer calories and without the detrimental side effects of inflammation. This is to say that they're wholly unnecessary.

- **Avoid processed/industrial oils.** Common vegetable and seed oils, such as cottonseed oil, safflower oil, sunflower oil, corn oil, peanut oil, and soybean oil, all require a considerable amount of processing to make them edible. Consequently, when many of these oils are exposed to light or heat, they quickly turn rancid. Rancid oils contain free radicals, are highly inflammatory, and sometimes taste weird. If you have any of these oils in your home, our advice is to promptly relocate them from your cupboard to your trash can.

Making the Paleo diet work for you

At first glance, the Paleo diet can seem a little intimidating. And we understand that you have to overcome many obstacles when getting started on a new nutritional regimen. But we assure you, the Paleo diet is both practical and reasonable. Furthermore, no other nutritional regimen guarantees such high performance or effective recovery from intense bouts of exercise.

Also, keep in mind that no fitness program, no matter how cleverly it's designed or how vehemently you adhere to it, is enough to ward off the harmful effects of poor eating habits.

And when you eat right — that is, when you eat like a cave man — you can expect four times the results from Paleo fitness than you could otherwise. So, it could also quite easily be said that when you eat poorly, you can expect one-fourth of the results.

Fat loss starts and ends in the kitchen. Exercise just hastens the process. A proper Paleo nutrition plan is crucial for your success.

We talk about Paleo nutrition extensively in Part IV, but we encourage you to pick up a copy of our sister book, *Living Paleo For Dummies* (Wiley). In there, you'll find everything you need to know about the Paleo diet and how to apply it to your everyday life.

Chapter 3

Running the Primal System Restore on Yourself

Humans are movers first, foremost, and forevermore. The cave man understood this and incorporated movement into his everyday life. His body and health benefited immensely from movement because movement is maintenance. It keeps the body young. And when you move, you thrive.

Although the human body is durable, it won't last forever. People won't always be able to move beautifully and lift heavy, but far too many fall apart far too soon. Sometimes, this deterioration is unavoidable, such as when disease or injury take hold, but often, people's bodies fail because of neglect.

Routine checkups and upkeep delays the steady, inevitable, and systematic decline. And although you may not be able to completely prevent dysfunction, disorder, and death, you can postpone it by doing what you can while you can. We show you how.

In this chapter, you find that restoring your body, posture, and movement takes just a few minutes of diligent practice a day.

Moving with Your Brain

The brain controls all movement (in fact, the original need for a human nervous system, from an evolutionary standpoint, was to coordinate movement). The brain contains hundreds of billions of neurons (cells), with each single neuron making thousands upon thousands of connections to other neighboring neurons. These neural connections are the circuitry that enables all activity — both mental and physical.

To illustrate this point, think of riding a bike for the first time. It likely felt clumsy and awkward. If you tried it without training wheels, you may have even fell onto the pavement (and probably more than once). Your brain worked hard to establish the neural pathways to enable you to perform this activity efficiently. But with enough practice, patience, and band-aids, the day finally came when riding a bike felt effortless. Finally, your brain hard-wired the neural pathway for this activity, everything coordinated efficiently, and the ride was smooth.

Functional and efficient movement relies on connections in the brain. For the most part, you hard-wire these connections throughout early development by crawling, rolling, rocking, and eventually walking. You're designed to move beautifully, so it's part of your natural circuitry. However, the brain, like other muscles, follows a use-it-or-lose-it principle. When you challenge your brain, it has the ability to adapt — to create new neurons and new neural connections. But when you neglect your brain, these connections may break down. Over time, you may lose your ability to move functionally.

The more you move, the more you feed the brain, and the stronger the infrastructure becomes. You could even go so far as to think of movement as the ultimate brain-enhancing drug — it stimulates the growth of new cells and keeps the brain biologically young.

In the next sections, we explain the consequences of not moving and introduce the benefits of incorporating movement throughout the day, every day.

How movement affected evolution

Strong evidence suggests that humans are intelligent creatures due in large part to our movement history. Brains were once believed to be shaped by social interaction, eating meat, and the need to think, but now many scientists and anthropologists believe that our brains were shaped largely by movement and physical activity.

Studies show that all movement and physical activity leads to higher levels of substances in the human body proven to enhance performance and stimulate the brain. One of these substances is known as *brain-derived neurotrophic factor*, or BDNF.

So what can you get from all of this? Well, knowing the impact of movement on the brain helps you understand that movement leads to greater abilities — mentally and otherwise. And movement is not only primal but also essential to your development and overall well-being.

Understanding the consequences of stillness

Stillness, or a lack of physical activity, has many potential consequences, such as the following:

- ✔ Cardiovascular disease
- ✔ Depression
- ✔ Increased risk of injury
- ✔ Loss of bone density (higher risk for osteoporosis)
- ✔ Muscular atrophy (the weakening of muscles)
- ✔ Obesity
- ✔ Poor self-image
- ✔ Sleep apnea

There's no such thing as a wrong movement. You can suffer only from a lack of or underprepared movement.

A lack of movement is like a drought of sunshine, water, or food. Movement is as essential to your livelihood as good soil is to the health of a plant. Unfortunately, modern conveniences, such as cars, elevators, and escalators, have replaced much of the need for frequent, low-intensity movement.

One possible solution to combat these "conveniences" is to reject them and revert to a truly Paleolithic lifestyle. But doing so would surely flip you over the edge of reason and make for an unnecessarily difficult life. Can you imagine having to club your dinner to death every night?

Instead, we propose a more reasonable alternative: short bouts of movement performed intermittently throughout the day.

Aging gracefully with movement

Movement is the ultimate antiaging supplement for both your body and your brain. Best of all, movement is cumulative, meaning that small movements performed throughout the day are just as effective, if not more effective, than performing all of your movement at one time. The same goes for exercise, too!

The primal movements we suggest demand little time, effort, or equipment. All you have to do is remember to do them. Most of the movements we introduce in this chapter involve rolling, crawling, and rocking. We chose these movements for the following reasons:

✔ They're specifically designed to stimulate the brain in a developmental fashion (by mimicking how babies first learn to move) and, therefore, restore functional movement.

✔ They make for fun and effective warm-ups before exercise.

Prepping Your Body for Primal Movement

In this section, you discover how to hack into your neurological hard-wiring and press the system reset button to restore the beautiful movement programming of your youth.

The following primitive movements are designed to carve out (or re-carve) the neural pathways (the connections in your brain) that allow for beautiful, functional, and efficient movement. These movements challenge and improve reflexive stability (both dynamic and static), motor control, and mobility.

You'll quickly discover that these movements are designed to improve *proprioception* — your awareness of self or sense of relative position in space — to provide the brain with the information it needs to re-establish functional movement patterns.

Proprioception is a sort of communication system within your body. Clear communication between the systems in your body results in functional movement, whereas muddled communication results in dysfunctional movement. The aim of these exercises is to improve the communication system.

And because the largest proprioceptive organ in your body is your skin, don't be surprised to find that many of these movements start you out on the ground (lots of surface area contact with the skin) and are quite similar to those that babies first use to earn their authentic and beautiful movement.

The Turkish get-up

If we're ever exiled and allowed to take with us only one exercise to preserve ourselves, we'd take the Turkish get-up. This primitive exercise has you moving from just about every joint in your body, forcing you to stabilize where you need to stabilize and mobilize where you need to mobilize. Its primary purpose is to get you up off the ground safely.

Furthermore, this movement is the most comprehensive of all primal warm-ups. Five minutes of consecutive Turkish get-ups will prep the body for any and all rigors of vigorous exercise.

You can perform the Turkish get-up anywhere, anytime. To keep on the move and to reap the maximum benefit of this exercise, we recommend that you set yourself a daily Turkish get-up quota. Try working even just one unweighted Turkish get-up every hour you're awake. You'll be amazed at how refreshing it feels!

The Turkish get-up — or *get-up* for the sake of brevity — toughens the shoulders, hardens the abs, and loosens the hips through an exhibition of litheness. It's a graceful movement with many nuances.

Don't rush the get-up. In fact, the slower you go, the better. Take time to master each position and enjoy the ride.

A proper setup for the get-up is essential; an improper setup impedes the crusade downstream, which is to say that any get-up is only as good as any setup. *Note:* When first performing the get-up, don't use any weight. After you're proficient at the movement, you may then use a kettlebell (preferred), a dumbbell (second best), or a barbell (most awkward but doable).

Here are the steps for the Turkish get-up:

1. **Start by lying on your back (prone position).**

   Your arms and legs should be fully extended and angled out away from your body at roughly 45 degrees. Your right arm should run parallel to your right leg and your left arm parallel to your left leg. Think of the bottom of a snow angle position.

2. **Pick a side to start with, follow these steps, and refer to Figure 3-1 to continue the setup:**

   a. To work the right side of your body, press your right arm directly up in line with your sternum (mid-chest) as if you're performing a one-arm bench press.

   b. Bend your right knee and plant your right heel relatively (not directly) close to your butt.

   Note: To work on the left side, follow the steps with your left arm and left leg.

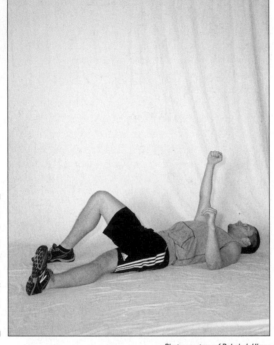

Photo courtesy of Rebekah Ulmer

3. **Perform a roll by pushing hard into your planted heel, pulling hard from your planted elbow, driving your chest upward, and propping yourself up onto your planted forearm (see Figure 3-2a).**

   Keep your other arm extended straight overhead (imagine you're balancing a half cup of water on your fist at all times — don't let it spill!).

   This step is to be a roll, not a crunch or a sit-up. If you lead with your head and round your back, then you're doing it wrong. Lead with a proud chest, and keep your back flat.

4. **Move from your forearm up to your hand by extending the elbow (see Figure 3-2b).**

   Don't lift your hand to do this step; instead, simply pivot on it. An effective, but somewhat crude, cue is to pretend you're squishing a beetle. Also, don't let your shoulders shrug up in this position. Keep as much distance between your shoulders and ears as possible.

5. **Complete a bridge by pushing your heel into the ground, squeezing your butt, and driving your hips up into the air (see Figure 3-3a).**

   Try your very best to come into a full bridge, but don't overextend. You should be able to freely lift your straight leg off the ground in the bridge position. If you can't, you need to shift your weight onto the heel of your bent leg.

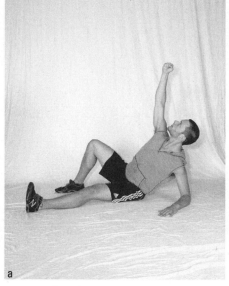 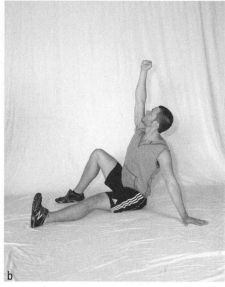

Figure 3-2:
Start the get-up by performing a roll (a) and then moving to your hand (b).

a

b

Photos courtesy of Rebekah Ulmer

6. **Sweep your straight leg back under your hips, planting your knee directly in line with your planted hand (see Figure 3-3b).**

   When done right, your legs should form an *L* with one knee facing forward and the other knee facing outward.

   Don't try to sweep your leg back in such a manner that both knees face forward, like they would in a lunge position. Doing so feels awkward and will put you into a bad position.

7. **Simultaneously lift your planted hand and rotate your back leg to come up off the ground and into an overhead lunge position (see Figure 3-4a).**

   The movement of your back leg should look similar to a windshield wiper as your back calf swings outward until both knees are pointed in the same direction.

8. **Stand up out of the lunge, as shown in Figure 3-4b.**

   Note that in the lunge position (Step 7), you want your back toes to be firmly planted on the ground (not pointed behind you) so you can push off your back leg just as much as your front leg to stand up.

9. **Reverse everything you just did — step by step — and return to the starting position.**

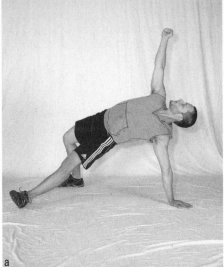
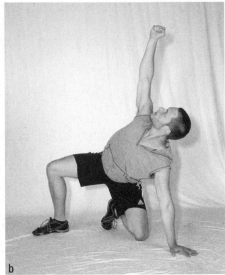

Figure 3-3:
Push into
the bridge
position (a)
and then the
sweep (b).

a

b

Photos courtesy of Rebekah Ulmer

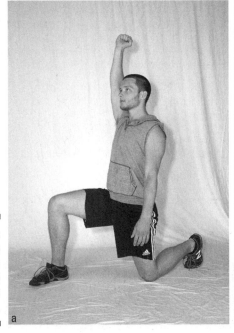
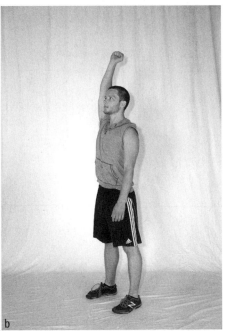

Figure 3-4:
Move to
a lunge
position (a)
and then
stand up (b).

a

b

Photos courtesy of Rebekah Ulmer

Practice the get-up as often as you can and get comfortable with it because you'll use it in other movements throughout this book. Eventually, you'll load the get-up and execute it with a considerable amount of weight overhead, enhancing your strength, stability, mobility, and coordination.

Rolling

As we mention earlier in this chapter, *proprioception,* or the awareness of your body position, ties all the senses together. High proprioception allows you to move skillfully without thinking about it. Low proprioception, however, results in awkward and often dysfunctional movement.

Proprioception is supported partly by the vestibular system, which coordinates your movement through changes in head position. You garner information about your position through all your senses — seeing, feeling, hearing, smelling, and so forth.

Those with low proprioception are often undersensitized to changes in position; hence, their body doesn't react accordingly, and they move clumsily, putting them at a higher risk for injury.

Because skin is the largest sensory organ on the body, movements designed to increase the surface area contact between skin and the ground — like rolling — will likely improve proprioception. In other words, the more time you spend on the ground, the better your movement will be off the ground.

From a developmental standpoint, you can't regress movement any farther back than rolling, nor does any movement put you into as much contact with the ground. So rolling is one of the best movements to improve proprioception and to prep the body for the rigors of exercise.

Here, we cover four types of simple rolling:

✔ **Rolling from your back onto your stomach from your upper body:**

1. Lie flat on your back with your legs and arms fully extended. Imagine that you're paralyzed from the waist down.

2. To roll to one side, slowly reach across and down your body with your opposite arm almost as if you're trying to reach something in your opposite pocket (see Figure 3-5).

   For example, to roll to your right side, reach across with your left arm. To roll to your left, reach with your right arm.

3. Continue to reach with your arm, head, and shoulders until you achieve lift and are able to flip yourself onto your stomach without any assistance from the lower body.

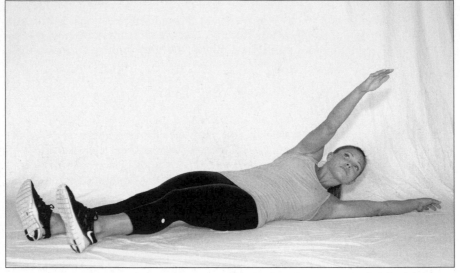

Figure 3-5:
When rolling from your top half, let your head and arm guide the motion.

Photo courtesy of Rebekah Ulmer

✔ **Rolling from your stomach onto your back from your upper body:**

1. Lie flat on your stomach with your legs and arms fully extended. Imagine that you're paralyzed from the waist down.

2. To roll to one side, slowly turn your head to your opposite side and attempt to look behind you as far as you can. Simultaneously reach your arm up and as far back behind you as possible.

   For example, to roll to your right side, turn your head to the left and reach your left arm up. To roll to your left, turn to the right and reach up with your right arm.

3. Continue to lead with your head and reach back with your arm until you're able to flip yourself onto your back without any assistance from your lower body.

In this case, the body follows the head. If you get stuck when attempting to roll from your upper body, you may not be looking or leading enough with the head.

✔ **Rolling from your back onto your stomach from your lower body:**

1. Lie flat on your back with your arms and legs fully extended. Imagine that you're paralyzed from the waist up.

2. To roll to one side, reach your knee up and across your body until your hips begin to lift and you're able to flip yourself onto your stomach without any assistance from your upper body (see Figure 3-6).

   For example, to roll to your right side, reach up with your left knee. To roll to your left, reach up with your right knee.

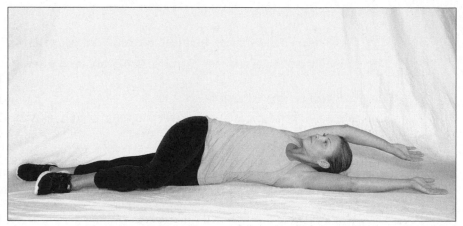

Figure 3-6:
When roll-
ing from
your bottom
half, let your
leg and hips
control the
movement.

Photo courtesy of Rebekah Ulmer

✔ **Rolling from your stomach onto your back from your lower body:**

1. Lie flat on your stomach with your arms and legs fully extended. Imagine that you're paralyzed from the waist up.

2. To roll to one side, reach your leg back and across your body until your hips begin to lift and you're able to flip yourself onto your back without any assistance from your upper body.

   For example, to roll to your right side, reach your left leg back. To roll to your left, reach your right knee back.

You shouldn't have to use any momentum when rolling. Perform this movement in a slow-reaching manner, like how a baby would do it.

Crawling

Simple crawling movements loosen the hips, prime the core, and warm up the shoulders. Crawling also ties your movement together; it syncs the right and left hemispheres of your brain through *contralateral movement* — the movement of corresponding body parts on opposite sides, such as moving your right arm and left leg together and vice versa.

Humans are naturally contralateral movers. This means that when you walk, you ought to move your left arm with your right leg and your right arm with your left leg. Crawling can help reset these natural contralateral patterns, which, in turn, reduces your risk of injury.

And depending on how you serve it, crawling, just like the Turkish get-up, makes for a great workout in and of itself. In fact, it's a marvelous cardiovascular and metabolic conditioning exercise.

The two variations of crawling are

- Crawling on hands, knees, and feet, forward, backward, and sideways
- Crawling on hands and feet, forward, backward, and sideways

On your hands, knees, and feet

Crawling on your hands, knees, and feet is often referred to as *creeping*. You want to start with creeping because it provides a larger base of support, and you perform it in a slower manner. Simple creeping works wonders for the hips, shoulders, and core.

To set up for creeping, get down on your hands and knees, and place your arms directly under your shoulders and your knees directly under your hips. Your feet should be planted, not pointed — meaning your toes are tucked. Keep your back flat at all times. Refer to Figure 3-7 and then follow these steps to crawl forward, backward, and sideways:

1. **Move forward by moving your opposite arm and leg together.**

   Your right arm should move with your left leg, and your left arm should move with your left leg.

2. **Move backward by simply reversing the movement of Step 1.**

3. **Creep laterally, or sideways, by matching the movement of your right arm to your left leg and vice versa.**

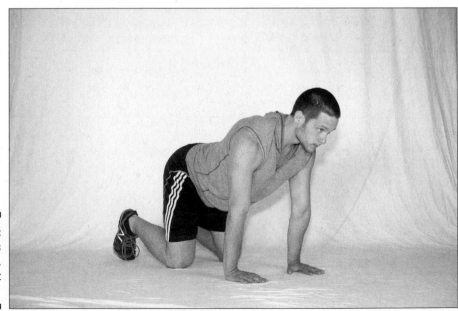

Figure 3-7:
Creeping is child's play, literally, but it's no joke!

Photo courtesy of Rebekah Ulmer

On just your hands and feet

After you feel like you have a good handle on creeping, you may progress to crawling on just your hands and feet, also known as *bear crawls.* To set up for crawling, get down on your hands and knees, and place your hands directly under your shoulders and your knees directly under your hips. Then lift your knees slightly off the ground and turn your hands and feet slightly outward if that feels more comfortable. (See Figure 3-8.) Your knees should remain bent and your butt relatively low. Then follow these steps to move forward, backward, and sideways:

1. **Move forward the same way you would with creeping, by matching up your opposite arm and leg.**

2. **Reverse the movement from Step 1 to crawl backward.**

3. **Move to your left and right, following the instructions for the creeping exercise.**

Take five minutes right now to get down on the ground and crawl around. Try crawling forward, backward, left and right. It may seem tricky or awkward at first, but keep practicing. Over time, crawling will feel more and more fluid.

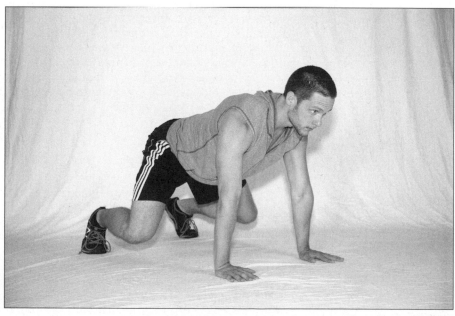

Figure 3-8: When crawling, feel free to play around with your head position, looking down between your hands or slightly up toward the horizon.

Photo courtesy of Rebekah Ulmer

Avoiding Injury: What to Do Before and After Exercise

Ever wonder what you should do immediately before and after exercise? The answer, our friends, is to move. Injury is largely the result of movement dysfunction, asymmetries, restrictions, and, well, general stupidity. Crawling, rolling, and Turkish get-ups (all of which we talk about in the previous section) will help with the first three. As for the last one, all we can do is set forth the following rule: *If something doesn't feel right, don't do it!*

Don't ever go into pain when exercising. Don't ever go into pain when moving. Don't ever go into pain, ever. The only place you should go when you have pain is the doctor's.

If you were a cave man constantly on the move, you wouldn't need to prep your body before any vigorous activity, because as a creature that lives dynamically, you'd always be ready for exertion. A lion, too, for example, doesn't need to stretch before sprinting and tackling its prey because the lion is always ready.

People, today, however, are far removed from the cave man or the lion. People, on average, sit more than they stand, and a hunt usually involves little more than shimmying through the cafeteria lunch line. Therefore, for your own safety, take time (ten minutes is usually plenty) before (and after) each training session to explore movement and to prep your body for exercise.

In the following sections, we outline what you must know and must do before and after exercise (and what you can do without).

Preparing before exercise

Don't get terribly excited about stretching before exercising or horribly upset if you skip stretching before exercise altogether. It's not that big of a deal, especially if you've been on the move regularly and have taken at least five minutes or so to practice crawling, rolling, and/or Turkish get-ups (see the earlier section "Prepping Your Body for Primal Movement").

Not too many people truly get all that flexible through stretching anyway, and strong evidence suggests that prolonged static stretching before exercise may inhibit your ability to perform optimally. Muscle suppleness, like movement, is linked to the nervous system; in other words, it's your ability to relax. Rarely will yanking at muscles improve your long-term flexibility, because rarely does such a practice promote a state of relaxation.

The key to flexibility is to stretch gently at first and to discover how to relax yourself into a greater range of motion. Be patient and let it come — don't force it.

Relaxing after exercise

Although your priority should always be to improve movement quality, gentle stretching after exercise can still be beneficial.

When stretching after exercise (and even before), go to the beginning of the stretch and hold it there, whatever the stretch may be. Hold it for as long as it takes for you to feel relaxed, to comfortably move into a deeper range of motion. This could take 30 seconds, 10 minutes, or it may not even happen at all. Don't worry about it. Just don't push too far too soon; otherwise, you'll tense up and defeat the purpose of the stretch, which is to train your body to relax into a greater range of motion.

Part II
Mastering the Primal Power Moves

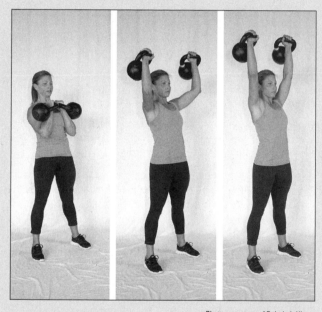

Photos courtesy of Rebekah Ulmer

For more tips on performing kettlebell exercises, check out www.dummies.com/extras/paleoworkouts.

In this part . . .

- ✔ Forgo the jog and start walking and sprinting for fat loss and muscle building.

- ✔ Progress through exercises to develop lower body strength and discover why lower body strength is so important for your overall health and fitness.

- ✔ See why your body weight alone is a powerful tool for developing upper body strength, and get familiar with the best exercises that use traditional weights to create lean, hardened, and healthy chest, back, and shoulders.

- ✔ Forget the crunches and sit-ups and develop a lean, strong core by simply carrying weight.

- ✔ Take your training to the next level with advanced, power-developing exercises, such as the push press, jerk, and double snatch.

Chapter 4

Walk to Get Healthy, but Sprint to Get Sexy

In This Chapter

▶ Discovering how frequent, slow movement nourishes the body

▶ Identifying when and how often to "run for your life"

One of the starkest differences between the lifestyle of the cave man and people today is movement frequency. Our ancestors spent more time on their feet than they did their butts. Today that trend is reversed entirely, and it has done a lot of harm.

The cave man moved about often pursuing the necessities of life. The majority of his movement was slow walking, but moving so regularly at a relatively low intensity is in large part what kept the cave man so lean and healthy.

On the other end of the force-velocity spectrum, the cave man, at times, had to run like his life depended on it, which in some situations, it really did! This combination of frequent slow moving and occasional bouts of all-out sprinting is a potent means for total body leanness, power, and vitality.

In this chapter, we show you how to best combine slow and fast primal movements to maximize leanness and well-being and how to apply these movements to a modern lifestyle.

Walking: Low-Intensity Movement for Health

When we say *walking,* we really mean any low-intensity movement that keeps you between 50 to 75 percent of your maximum heart rate. Exercising at this intensity, you can still comfortably hold a conversation.

Don't worry about a heart rate monitor. If you already have one, feel free to use it. But as long as you're moving slow without any huffing or puffing, you're probably right where you need to be.

In this section, we explore the benefits of moving slowly, at a walking pace, and show you how to incorporate those movements into all areas of your life. We also provide a skill drill for walking to help you get the most out of low-intensity movements.

Recognizing the benefits of moving slowly and often

Don't discount low-intensity exercise on the premises of difficulty. Just because it doesn't leave you gasping for air or your body flushed with lactic acid doesn't mean it isn't doing you any good. In fact, when performed regularly, low-intensity exercise may have the most positively profound impact on your overall health than any other form of exercise.

Here are a few benefits of frequent, low-intensity exercise:

- ✔ Counteracts the hormonal effects of stress
- ✔ Reduces your risk of metabolic syndrome and diabetes
- ✔ Reduces your risk of heart disease and cancer
- ✔ Decreases overall inflammation
- ✔ Burns fat while preserving muscle
- ✔ Improves your mood

Finding the time for walking and hiking

When starting out on your primal fitness journey, we encourage you to incorporate at least seven hours of low-intensity physical activity each week. Preferably, one hour every day. The possibilities of low-intensity activities reach far beyond what we can include in one book, so we give you a few of our favorites and leave the rest to your imagination.

If you're going to start anywhere, simple walking and hiking is as good a place as any. The cave man did it, and so should you.

The best time to perform low-intensity physical activity is in the morning hours before your first meal. Fasted walking is a technique people have used for thousands of years to stay super lean and healthy. The fact is, when you wake up, your body is already in a condition primed for fat-burning, so take advantage of that and add in some early morning low-intensity walking before breakfast.

You don't have to do all your low-intensity physical activity at one time. Feel free to break it up throughout the day. Activity and exercise is cumulative. Try a half hour in the morning before breakfast and a half hour at night before dinner.

Doing what you love

With low-intensity exercise, it doesn't really matter *how* you do it, just that you do it. The adherence to the activity, not necessarily the activity itself, weighs heaviest on your success.

To this end, we encourage you to seek out low-intensity activities that you enjoy. When you love what you do, you do a better job at it and do it more often than if you're forced into something that leaves you feeling bored, indifferent, or annoyed. From chasing the kids, to water sports, from golfing, to Frisbee, to skiing, the movement possibilities are endless. And that's all we're after — more movement. What you do doesn't matter so long as you stay on the move. Just don't exert yourself too much. We save that for later (when we talk about high-intensity exercise).

Your low-intensity physical activity should keep you at about 55 to 70 percent of your maximum heart rate. Don't worry about getting a heart rate monitor. If you aren't huffing or puffing, you're probably doing all right.

Moving often but living slow

Even though the focus of this chapter is movement, it's also important to slow things down a bit — not necessarily your movement but your mind.

Staying on the move doesn't mean living fast; it means living active. Moving often but living slow is an art, and it takes practice. Slowing your mind and taking the time to meditate, breathe, and appreciate are as equally essential to your health as movement is.

Slow, frequent moving helps with this process. Outdoor hiking, walking, and other such leisurely activities gives you permission to take it all in, to savor it, and to calm your mind.

Living slow, like almost anything else, is a choice. It's a choice to connect with the world and with others on a deeper level. It's a choice to do less and to unshackle the mind from unnecessary distractions.

Here are a few other things to start taking a bit more slowly:

- **Breathing:** Employ a deeper, slower breath whenever you can. Doing so will help control stress and alleviate tension.
- **Eating:** Take the time to enjoy each bite. Resist the urge to gorge. Eating more slowly will also help you feel fuller quicker, which is a good thing.
- **Playing:** Strive to appreciate play like a kid again. Keep your focus in the present, and just be in the moment.
- **Having sex:** That's right, we said it. Slowing down in the bedroom will help you appreciate the experience more and make it more intimate.
- **Spending time with friends and family:** Take as much time as you can, while you can. Appreciate your friends and family now.
- **Traveling:** Whenever possible, travel by foot, and enjoy the journey. And it's okay to walk just to walk, because you enjoy walking — you don't always have to be going somewhere.

Slow living quite regularly leads to a more balanced life, less stress, and a deeper sense of fulfillment.

Walking skill drill: Marching

This section provides you with a simple drill to help you improve your walking technique. You can, and should, practice this drill nearly every day.

You may be thinking, *why do I need to practice walking?* Well, the truth is, most people fake walking — that is, they don't have proper walking mechanics. The skill drill of marching helps reset your natural *contralateral* walking pattern. Contralateral simply means opposite limb movement, matching your right arm with your left leg and vice versa.

For example, when walking, you should gently sway your left arm forward as you step with your right foot. At just about all times, your opposite arms and legs should run parallel to each other.

Marching, shown in Figure 4-1, allows you to exaggerate and to reset this contralateral pattern. Here's how to do it:

1. **Stand tall with your feet approximately shoulder-width apart.**

2. **Bend your elbows to 90 degrees.**

3. **Simultaneously drive your right knee and left elbow upward and toward your center line.**

4. **Touch your right knee and left elbow together at or around belly height, pause momentarily, and bring them both back to the starting position.**

5. **Repeat the pattern with your left knee and right elbow.**

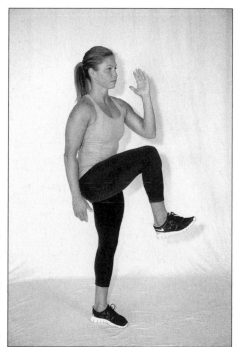

Figure 4-1:
Marching
helps reset
your natural
walking
pattern.

Photo courtesy of Rebekah Ulmer

Practice this drill stationary at first (in one place) then start to move with it.

Sprinting: High-Intensity Movement for Physique

Sprinting is the most potent thing in the world for building muscle and shedding fat. The form of a sprinter is that of a classic, powerful physique. Lean, dense, hard. Built for speed and grace.

The cave man was an avid sprinter. He had to be. He ran to eat and to not be eaten. So sprinting not only kept the cave man alive but also attributed to his overall leanness and muscularity.

In the following sections, we lay out the benefits of moving with high-intensity, at a sprinting pace, and give you the lowdown on how to do so, how much (or how far), and how often. We also provide a skill drill for sprinting to keep your form powerful and graceful.

Discovering the benefits of high-speed movement

The benefits of sprinting are so numerous and profound that a simple list of bullet points hardly seems to do it a full service, but here are a few of the highlights:

- Builds muscle (unlike jogging or other forms of moderate-intensity cardio)
- Surges growth hormone
- Blasts fat
- Causes a huge metabolic response and caloric after-burn
- Develops explosive power
- Improves ability to ward off fatigue
- Doesn't take long

Running for your life

You should approach sprinting as an art to be practiced and nothing else. It's not something to be thrown around loosely. Sprinting, when done right (and when done at the right times), ignites the metabolic furnace and triggers the muscle-building machinery. When done wrong, or when horribly overworked, it's potentially injurious.

Properly preparing your body for the rigors of sprinting is imperative. This exercise is a super high-velocity movement, so don't go into it cold. Strides, which we discuss in the "Sprinting skill drill: Strides" section, are one way to prime the body for sprinting. Whatever you do, just be sure to ease your way into an all-out sprint.

Here are the elements of proper sprinting mechanics to strive for (see Figure 4-2):

✔ Heel has minimal contact with the ground.

✔ Foot strikes the ground roughly under the hips.

✔ Torso remains fairly upright and stays at the same height throughout the sprint.

✔ Elbows stay at 90 degrees.

✔ Shoulders (not elbows) initiate arm swing.

✔ Movement of the arms match the movement of the legs in a contralateral fashion (arm rises and falls with opposite leg).

If, for whatever reason, sprinting on foot isn't for you, try bike sprints. Bike sprints are similar to running sprints in that you try to move as quickly as possible, basically going all out as you pedal the bike. You can use a stationary bike or a regular one if you prefer. Although bike sprints aren't as beneficial as running sprints, they allow for a lower impact variation of sprinting.

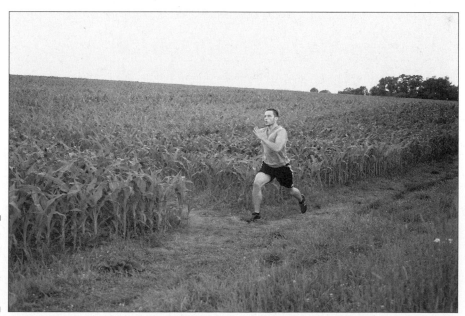

Figure 4-2: Sprinting is about blending power with grace.

Photo courtesy of Rebekah Ulmer

Sprinting may feel awkward at first, especially if you haven't done it in a while. But, as with all other forms of movement, the more you practice, the better you'll get. Treat sprinting as practice instead of a workout. The sweat will come, but let it be the consequence of diligent rehearsal, not mindless running for running's sake.

Practicing sprints for power and grace

So how far and how long should you sprint? Well, the answer, as any good strength coach will tell you, is that it depends.

Don't worry too much about distance at first. The goal is to run as powerfully and as gracefully as possible — not to run for as long or as far as possible. To this end, pick a distance long enough for you to express power but short enough to maintain good form. You may be able to go only a very short distance at first, and that's okay. As you continue to practice and as your body conditions, you can expand the distance and shorten the rest periods.

How often should you sprint? Again, that depends. But generally, when starting out, you should sprint once every week or once every two weeks.

 When sprinting, set a timer for 10 to 15 minutes and just practice. Rest as long as you need to catch your breath and freshen up for the next set. As you become more proficient and better conditioned, you can then increase the distance (or time) and shorten the rest periods.

Sprinting skill drill: Strides

Sprinting, like all other movement, is a skill. But because sprinting is such a high-velocity movement, it merits a little extra consideration than most other movements. Proper sprinting prep and mechanics can mean the difference between a fantastic workout and a torn hamstring.

The skill drill for this section focuses on strides. *Strides* are a popular running technique that can only be described as something between a jog and a sprint. They help you prep the body for sprints and rehearse proper sprinting mechanics.

Strides are best performed barefoot and on an unpaved surface (try working them on the soccer field at a community park, but be sure the field is well kept so you don't land in a divot and injur yourself).

Check out Figure 4-3 to see what strides look like, and refer to the following list on how to perform strides:

✔ Perform strides in a similar fashion to a sprint workout (six to eight rounds of 60 to 100 meters), but feel free to adjust the distance as needed.

When you start, gradually accelerate to about 85 percent of your max speed for the first two-thirds and then gradually decelerate in the final one-third of the stride.

✔ Focus on form as you do strides. Ensure a quick foot turnover, striking the ground on the ball of your foot in line with your hip (don't overstride).

✔ Think "quick arms" on the stride, and match the pumping of your arms to the pumping of your legs.

Just like marching (discussed earlier in this chapter), strides should be a contralateral movement, meaning your opposite arm and leg move together — that is, when your left leg rises, so does your right arm, and vice versa.

✔ Maintain a fairly upright torso.

Keep in mind that strides aren't supposed to be difficult. Don't do them at such a fast pace that your warm-up becomes as strenuous as your workout. Strides are drills, not sprints.

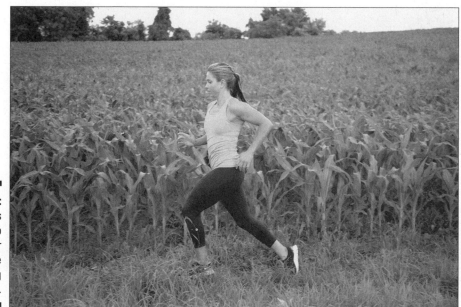

Figure 4-3:
Use strides to prep yourself for an intense sprinting session.

Photo courtesy of Rebekah Ulmer

Chapter 5

Hinging and Squatting Your Butt and Legs to Primal Perfection

● ●

In This Chapter

▶ Developing hinge movements

▶ Discovering how to squat deeply (without wrecking your knees)

▶ Mastering progressions to improve your lower body strength and mobility

● ●

*I*n terms of neuromuscular activation, squats and hinges soar high above most other exercises; they recruit more muscle fibers, demand more metabolically, and subsequently chop more fat and build more muscle.

To keep it simple, you can think of hinging as maximum hip bend with some knee bend, and you can think of squatting as maximum hip bend *and* knee bend. In a hinge, the butt reaches back. In a squat, the butt reaches down. Knowing the difference is important because hinges are heavily driven by the posterior chain (hamstrings, butt, lower back), whereas squats require a bit more from the anterior chain (front side), specifically, the quads.

This chapter is dedicated to showing you the primal hinging and squatting movements you need to form, firm, and strengthen the legs, butt, and midsection. Here, you discover how to perform the choicest lower body exercises for a cast-iron posterior and legs that won't quit — all without wrecking your knees or wrenching your back.

The Lowdown on Hinges

The purpose of the hinge is to move and produce force from the hips. This is a necessarily life skill. Being able to move properly from the hips allows you to lift weight safely up off the ground without wrecking your back and maximizes your athletic abilities.

The most basic, or primal, hinging pattern is the dead lift: a bending of the hips to reach down and pick something up. Conventional wisdom tells you that you shouldn't lift with your back, but we say you *should* lift from your back — as well as from the rest of your posterior chain.

For example, when you watch a baby pick something up off the ground, the baby almost invariably reverts to the dead lift to do so. Very rarely will any baby pick something up from a squat because the dead lift (which we use interchangeably with *hinge* in this book) is the natural human crane position. When the back is kept flat, the hips reach back, and the knees bend slightly, you're in a position to heave a considerable load from the floor.

 Perhaps the most potentially injurious way to lift any weight off the ground, especially if you're new to weight training, is to do so with a rounded (hunched) back. When hinging, push your chest up (think "proud chest") to maintain the natural curvature of your spine.

The following sections give you a few more details and benefits about the hinge.

Using your hips in the hinge

An athlete's power comes from the hips. Hinging shows you how to fully utilize the strength and power of your hips. Whether you aim to pick something up without wrecking your back or to jump across a creek without ruining your pants, using your hips will help you do just that.

In a properly hinged position, the hips take the load, not the back. (And often, the hinge is referred to as a *hip hinge*.) A proper hinge ensures optimum spinal alignment and transmission of force; that is, when you hinge properly, the hips do the heavy lifting and the back is kept safe. Here's how:

1. **Keep your back flat (never rounded or overarched).**
2. **Push your hips back as far as possible.**
3. **Allow your knees to bend slightly (but not so much that they come forward).**

   The bottom of a hinge should have your legs and torso looking like the less than sign (<).

 Everyone's hinge will look slightly different. As long as your shins are vertical, your back is flat, and your hips are above the knees (but below the shoulders), you're good to go!

Counting the benefits of a strong hinge

We can't stress enough the importance of developing the hinge movement pattern. A strong, patterned hinge makes all the heavy lifting of life easier. Literally.

But there's more to it than that. A strong hinge offers the following benefits as well:

- ✔ Less risk of back injury
- ✔ Less risk of knee injury
- ✔ More power and athletic ability
- ✔ A stronger, firmer butt
- ✔ A resilient, sturdy back
- ✔ Functional, durable hamstrings

Practice your hinge as often as possible. Whether you're picking up a pencil or 500 pounds, get those hips back and keep the back flat!

Beginner Hinging Exercises

You can express the hinge in many ways. But like most all other movements, you should start out slow with the basics. To introduce the hinge, we start with the basic dead lift. The dead lift, which is picking something up (and putting it back down), is as fundamental as it gets.

Don't let the unpretentious nature of this movement fool you. The dead lift will be a staple in all the primal fitness programs because it's a monstrous strength-building exercise; it allows you to load the system with more weight than just about any other movement.

In the following sections, we outline the pattern for the dead lift and the single-leg dead lift.

The dead lift

The dead lift is simply the hinge put to work. To get started practicing the dead lift, you need something to pick up. We recommend a kettlebell or a dumbbell to start out (eventually you'll move on to a set of kettlebells, dumb-bells, or a barbell). Most men can start out with a weight between 35 and 40 pounds and most women, between 18 and 25 pounds.

1. **Stand on top of the weight so it's positioned between your heels, assume a shoulder-width stance, and point your toes out slightly (between 10 and 20 degrees). (See Figure 5-1a.)**

2. **Push your hips back toward the wall behind you.**

   Imagine you're reaching your butt back for a bench that's just out of reach.

3. **Keep your back flat, but let your knees bend as you continue to reach your butt back as far as you possibly can without toppling backward.**

4. **When you hit maximum hip bend, grab hold of the weight and take a deep breath into your belly. (See Figure 5-1b.)**

   Be sure to keep the head and neck in line with the rest of your back as well. Focus your eyes on the ground slightly in front of you or onto the horizon where the wall meets the floor.

5. **Push your heels hard into the ground and stand up as quickly as possible. (See Figure 5-1c.)**

6. **Reverse the movement to set the weight back onto the floor. Don't round your back to set the weight down.**

   Be sure to start and finish the dead lift with good posture.

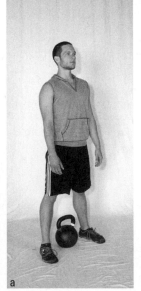 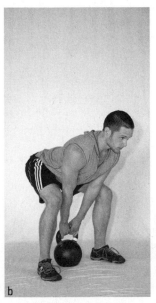 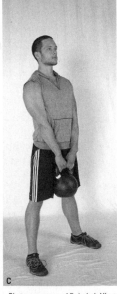

Figure 5-1:
The dead lift is the fundamental hinge movement.

a   b   c

Photos courtesy of Rebekah Ulmer

Whether you're lifting 35 pounds or 350, respect the weight all the same. Don't get into the habit of setting the weight down lazily or with poor form. What you practice is what you'll revert to when under stress. Get in the habit of doing it right.

If you're having trouble with the dead lift, check out these sections later in this chapter:

- ✔ If you're having trouble finding the proper hinge position or feel like you may be squatting the movement too much, see the section "The butt-to-wall drill."

- ✔ If you're having trouble keeping your back flat while hinging or feel like you may be overarching your back, see the section "The broomstick drill."

Sometimes mobility may be a limiting factor in the dead lift. If you feel like you have to compromise your form to reach down to the weight, bring the weight up to you! There's no point in performing an exercise unsuccessfully or with poor form when you can make small adjustments to help you train around mobility restrictions. Simply find a small box, or any other implement to elevate the weight, as shown in Figure 5-2, to make the weight easier to reach until your mobility improves.

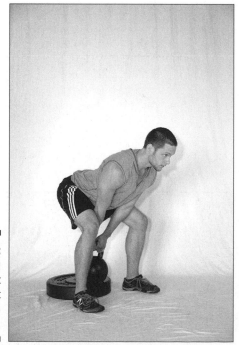

Figure 5-2:
Elevating the weight makes it easier to reach.

Photo courtesy of Rebekah Ulmer

The single-leg dead lift

The single-leg dead lift is pretty much what it sounds like — the dead lift using only one leg — with a few minor tweaks, of course. Most natural and athletic movements happen from a split stance, not an even one, so it's equally important to train the one-limbed (unilateral) movements as it is the two-limbed (bilateral) movements. The big benefits of the single-leg dead lift that don't necessarily come with the conventional dead lift are the additional balance, coordination, and motor control components.

We recommend using a kettlebell or dumbbell for this exercise, but if you want to develop extra balance and coordination, practice this movement as often as possible without weight. Here are the steps for the single-leg dead lift with a weight:

1. **Stand on top of the weight so it's positioned between your heels (refer to the setup for the dead lift in the previous section and see Figure 5-3a).**

2. **Push your heel back and up toward the ceiling.**

   Be sure to minimize any twisting and rotation throughout the movement. Both of your shoulders should fall and rise at the same rate; you want to keep them as square as possible throughout the movement.

3. **As your back heel starts to rise, naturally let yourself hinge at the hips.**

4. **Allow your knee to bend as you hinge.**

   To keep your balance, your knee may even come slightly forward in the single-leg dead lift.

   This is a single-leg dead lift. Not a "stiff leg" single-leg dead lift. So let the knee bend! If you don't, you run the risk of overloading the hamstring.

5. **When you're able to, reach down and grab the weight with the arm opposite the planted leg.**

   For example, if your right leg is on the ground, grab the weight with your left arm (see Figure 5-3b).

6. **Finish the movement the same way you came into it, standing tall at the top, as shown in Figure 5-3c.**

7. **Be sure to place the weight back down exactly how you picked it up.**

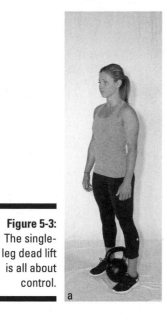
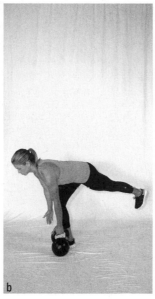
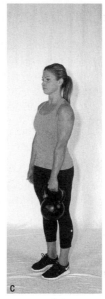

Figure 5-3:
The single-leg dead lift is all about control.

a   b   c

Photos courtesy of Rebekah Ulmer

Intermediate Hinging Exercises

The next step in hinging progressions is to add some power to the pattern. In this section, we introduce the swing and the one-arm swing, two explosive hinging exercises.

Don't proceed with intermediate hinging exercises prematurely. The swing is built off the back of the dead lift, so if you don't have that pattern close to perfect yet, your swing and everything else hereafter will suffer. If you need more practice with the dead lift, refer to the "Beginner Hinging Exercises" section.

Paleo fitness is about progressing at your own pace. There's no prize (at least that we know of) for being the first person to master all the exercises. The more time you spend practicing the basics, the easier the more advanced movements will be later on.

When you've mastered the dead lift, the swing comes easy, because the swing is really just a fast and continuous string of dead lifts.

The swing

Swings are as handy as hot sauce. They go well with anything and spice up even the blandest dishes. This is to say that you can pretty much add swings to any workout (foolishly assuming that you don't already do so) to instantly make it better.

The swing shows you how to generate power/explosiveness from your hips and is a marvelous all-around fat-chopping device. It blends strength and cardiovascular efforts, a trait shared by few exercises.

The swing also strengthens the muscles of the lower back, and strong evidence supports that swings may ward off back problems later in life. Swings also commonly lead to what has been affectionately dubbed the "kettlebutt" — a firm, strong, and aesthetically privileged backside.

We've found that the swing is best performed with a kettlebell (and it's often called a "kettlebell swing"), but you may use a dumbbell as well. A barbell is far too unwieldy for this exercise.

Here's how to do the swing:

1. **Assume a shoulder-width stance approximately one foot behind the weight you're using, and point your toes slightly outward.**

2. **Hinge at the hips like you would a dead lift (refer to the earlier section on the dead lift), reach out, and grab hold of the weight (see Figure 5-4a).**

   Be sure to get the hips back and keep the back flat.

3. **Start the swing with a forceful hike back of the weight, like a center hiking a football (see Figure 5-4b).**

   Keep the handle of the weight above your knees at all times; otherwise, your back may round. Also, don't be shy about the hike! You have to forcefully throw the weight back to properly load the hips for the swing.

4. **When the weight reaches the top of the backswing, immediately reverse the movement by driving your hips forward and standing up as quickly as you can.**

   Your hips and knees should extend simultaneously. Think "jump," but keep your heels planted on the ground. The hips should visibly snap forward when executing the swing. The aim is to be as explosive as possible, regardless of the weight you're using.

5. **Allow the weight to float no higher than eye level before reversing and repeating the movement. Don't lean back at the top of the swing; just stand tall. See Figure 5-4c.**

   If you have issues with your back, allow the weight to float no higher than shoulder level. When done right, the weight should float outward and upward. The movement is powered entirely by the hips. Your arms are simply loose chains connecting the weight to your body.

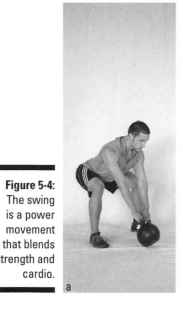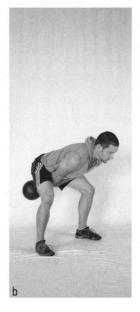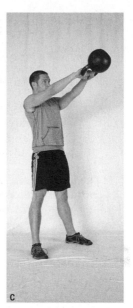

Figure 5-4: The swing is a power movement that blends strength and cardio.

a   b   c

Photos courtesy of Rebekah Ulmer

TIP While performing the swing, keep the arms relaxed but the armpits tight so your shoulders don't get pulled forward by the force of the weight. Imagine that you're squeezing a wad of cash or wringing a sponge in your armpit. This will help to keep the shoulders in a safely packed position.

The one-arm swing

The closest relative to the (two-arm/kettlebell) swing, the one-arm swing adds an additional grip challenge and rotary stability component (the ability to prevent rotation). Just like the two-arm swing, we recommend you use a kettlebell or dumbbell for this exercise.

Because you now bear the weight by only one side of the body, a good one-arm swing can be measured directly by the amount of rotation that doesn't occur. So do your very best to keep your shoulders square through the movement. Here are the steps to the one-arm swing:

1. **Set up like you would for a two-arm swing (see previous section), reach out, and grab the weight with one arm (see Figure 5-5a).**

   Grab the handle of the weight as close to dead center as possible.

2. **Hike the weight back as you would a two-arm swing while minimizing any twist in your torso (see Figure 5-5b).**

   With the one-arm swing, you may rotate your thumb slightly in (downward) on the backswing to ensure that the weight doesn't crash into the knees.

3. **When the weight reaches the top of the backswing, snap the hips forward and stand up as quickly as possible to complete the movement.**

4. **Allow the weight to float no higher than eye level (see Figure 5-5c) before reversing and repeating the movement.**

   If you have issues with your back, allow the weight to float no higher than shoulder level.

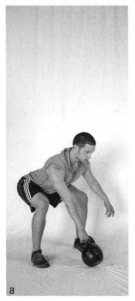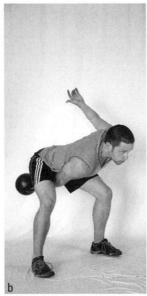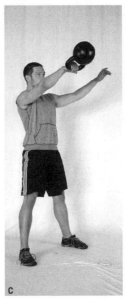

Figure 5-5: The one-arm swing.

Photos courtesy of Rebekah Ulmer

Remember to keep your armpit tight throughout the exercise. Don't let the weight pull your shoulder forward.

Advanced Hinging Exercises

In this section, we begin to tread less stable ground, both literally and metaphorically. These movements aren't more advanced in the sense that you perform them with more weight (although that may sometimes be the case) but because of the higher levels of control, concentration, and coordination required for proper execution.

For example, you wouldn't attempt the snatch before the two-arm swing any more than you'd ever try to juggle before first learning to catch.

With the beginner and intermediate hinging movements we introduce earlier in this chapter, we show you how to produce and reduce force from the hips — a necessary skill to maximize athletic potential and lessen injury risk. But there's one more skill you need to know, and that's the ability to redirect force — both toward you and away from you. To be able to both subtly and aggressively redirect force is a true exhibition of athleticism. You see this in all domains of sport; for example, the judo player who, through proper timing and subtle movement, redirects his opponent's oncoming force into a powerful hip toss.

But this is merely a hidden benefit. Cleans and snatches are markedly more infamous for building the back side, bolstering iron lung capacity, and butchering body fat.

The clean

The *clean,* another powerful hip-dominant movement, develops your ability to produce, reduce, and redirect force — a necessary athletic skill, even for non-athletes. The clean can also be a tremendous cardiovascular conditioner and power builder by itself. What's more is that heavy cleans, especially heavy double-kettlebell cleans, show you how to take a hit!

Cleans performed with a kettlebell or dumbbell differ slightly from cleans performed with barbells, sandbags, or other such devices that you can't easily swing between your legs. Here, we talk about kettlebell or dumbbell cleans because they're slightly more forgiving than barbell cleans (especially for those with restricted shoulder mobility), and the learning curve is less intimidating.

The purpose of the clean is to bring the weight explosively up into the rack position, where you place the weight in front of the chest so you can easily press, squat, jerk, and so on. In the rack, or the finished position of the clean, your forearms should be vertical and pressed against your rib cage. Here are the steps to the clean:

1. **Set up exactly how you would for a one-arm swing (see the earlier section), reach out, and grab the weight with one arm.**

2. **Start the clean with a forceful hike back of the weight (see Figure 5-6a).**

   Up until this point, the movement should be identical to the one-arm swing.

3. **When the weight reaches the top of the backswing, snap your hips forward (just like you would a swing).**

4. **As your hips drive forward, keep your elbow in close to your body and draw the weight up your center line (see Figure 5-6b).**

   Do your best to keep the weight as close to your body as possible. The more the weight casts outward, the less efficient the movement becomes. If it helps, imagine you're trying to zip up a big coat.

5. **Catch the weight in the rack position, with your forearm(s) against your rib cage, as shown in Figure 5-6c.**

   If you're using a kettlebell, allow it to gently roll onto the forearm before landing in the rack. A common mistake with the clean is to use the arms to curl the weight up. The hips must power the movement. Think about it like this: The hips are the engine, and the arm is the steering wheel.

Sometimes the best fix for poor clean technique is to pick up a heavier weight, which forces you to use more hips and less arms and to seek the most efficient trajectory. Most of the time, however, the best way to fix your clean is to go back and fix your swing and one-arm swing. The same goes for the snatch, which we talk about in the next section. Often, people venture into cleaning and snatching way too soon. Be sure to master the swing and one-arm swing before attempting the clean and the snatch; doing so will make the clean and the snatch that much easier.

Figure 5-6:
The clean starts like the one-arm swing and finishes in the rack position.

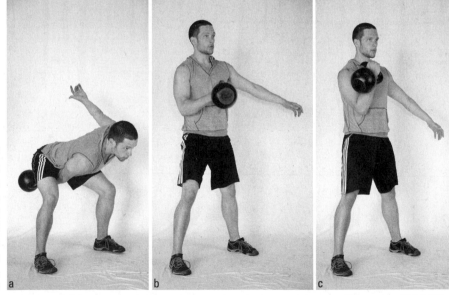

a   b   c

Photos courtesy of Rebekah Ulmer

The snatch

To perform the snatch, you swing the weight back between your legs and bring it up over your head in one smooth, uninterrupted motion. This movement brings you to the pinnacle of your primal hinging progressions.

The snatch builds on all the preceding exercises. If you haven't spent adequate time perfecting your swings, one-arm swings, and cleans, you're not ready for the snatch.

The snatch manufactures the raw power and "never say die" conditioning of an Olympian. And when applied liberally, it blasts body fat like a blowtorch. When you get into high-rep snatching, you'll see what we mean.

We focus primarily on kettlebell and dumbbell snatches because they're more forgiving, easier to learn, and don't require an Olympic lifting platform. Here's how to do the snatch:

1. **Set up behind the weight (kettlebell or dumbbell) like you would for a one-arm swing or clean (see earlier sections) and hike the weight forcefully back between your legs (see Figure 5-7a).**

2. **Drive your hips forward and explode out of the hinge. Imagine you're trying to jump through your heels.**

   To do the snatch right, you have to fully commit yourself to the movement; otherwise, the bell won't go where it needs to. Be sure to snap those hips!

3. **As the weight accelerates upward, keep your elbow in close to the body, guiding the weight up your center line (not letting it arch out wildly; see Figure 5-7b).**

   This portion of the snatch is sometimes referred to as the *high pull*. Notice in Figure 5-7b how the elbow is slightly bent and stays relatively in line with the body. This form ensures an efficient trajectory. The further the weight gets away from you on the way up, the less efficient the movement, so keep it tight.

4. **If using a kettlebell, practice "punching" through the bell around eye level to ensure a smooth transfer of the weight onto the forearm (see Figure 5-7c).**

   When you go to punch through the bell, be sure to loosen your grip to avoid tearing any callouses. It may even help if you "spear" through the bell and open your hand entirely.

5. **Finish the snatch overhead in a fully lockout position; that is, lock your elbow and line your bicep with or slightly behind your ear (see Figure 5-7d).**

It will take some time to find your groove, but in the end, the snatch should be one smooth and graceful movement.

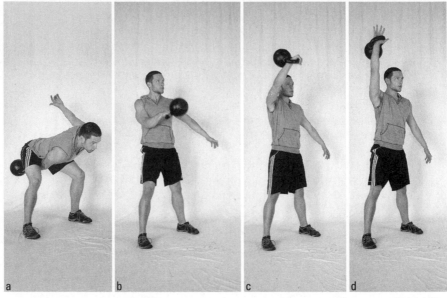

a   b   c   d

Figure 5-7:
The snatch is the pinnacle of primal hinging progressions.

Photos courtesy of Rebekah Ulmer

To avoid unnecessary callous tears when using kettlebells, maintain a relatively loose grip. Hold on just tight enough to keep the bell in your possession but loose enough so the handle may rotate without grinding up your hands.

The Lowdown on Squats

It's often joked that the squat is an essential movement for eating dinner in Thailand and taking care of business in the woods.

But there are other uses for the squat. The squat is the most potent of all exercises; pound for pound, it burns more calories and triggers more muscular activation than any other movement. The squat is also the king of all strength-building movements, and nothing can dethrone it.

Heavy squats are marvelous. They place a tremendous amount of stress on the body and flood the system with natural growth hormones (including natural human growth hormone).

Another benefit of the squat less talked about but equally valuable is to help you sit down, perhaps the most common application. But it should be noted that the original intention of this movement pattern was not to sit down but to stand up. People first enter the squat as babies, from the ground (often times out of a crawl) and use it to stand. So like the Turkish get-up (see Chapter 3), the squat is just as useful of a device to pick yourself up off the ground as it is to sit down onto it.

In the following sections, we squelch some common myths about squatting and explore the many benefits of this technique.

Getting to the truth about squatting

People often think squatting is bad for your knees. But we're here to tell you it isn't. *How* you squat may be bad for your knees, but the squat itself isn't bad for the knees. In fact, there are no bad movements, only a lack of preparation for movement. You need to strengthen the knees just like all other joints and muscles. And the only way to strengthen the knees is through movement.

If you have prior knee issues, or any issues for that matter, always get clearance from your doctor before beginning any type of fitness program.

Another common, somewhat silly myth, is that your knees shouldn't cross over your toes during a squat. We say it's okay if your knees cross over your toes as long as they stay in line with your toes. The knee is meant to bend. In fact, it's just about the only thing it can do, so let it do just that.

Exploring the benefits of a deep squat

The deep squat is an essential pattern. Ideally, you should be able to squat butt to ankles with your heels on the ground and your knees in line with your toes, all the while keeping your back relatively flat. Go ahead and give it a try! If you have the mobility, the bottom of a squat should feel like a rest position — like you could really hang out there for a while.

We imagine the cave man probably spent a lot of time hanging out in the bottom of a bodyweight squat, and we encourage you to do the same. The more time you can accumulate in the bottom of the squat throughout the day, the better. This position loosens your hips, toughens your joints, and gets you up off the couch!

As your deep squat improves, so will your lower body strength, lower body mobility, and general usefulness in society. An uninhibited squat is a strong indicator of functional movement. It requires ample mobility of the ankles, knees, and hips and stability of the pelvis. What does that mean? Well, a lot has to be working right for someone to squat deeply. It means your working equipment is somewhat in order, so you're less likely to fall apart.

Here are a few ways to work the squat into your daily routine:

- ✔ Answer at least ten e-mails a day from a squat.
- ✔ Talk on the phone from a squat.
- ✔ Watch TV from a squat (or, at the very least, watch the commercials from a squat).
- ✔ Eat one time during the day from a squat.
- ✔ When waiting in line, get down into a squat (let 'em stare!).

Beginner Squatting Exercises

The beginner squatting exercises that we introduce in this section are easy to understand and easy to use. They include the goblet squat, the bodyweight squat, and the goblet lunge. These squats are the most user-friendly variations; all intend to produce a big calorie burn while improving your squatting pattern.

Be patient with the squat, and don't get discouraged if you can't squat very low at first. The depth will come — especially when you combine the movements in Chapter 3 with the squatting skill drills later in this chapter. And don't ever push into a range of motion where you feel uncomfortable or are unable to maintain proper form.

The goblet squat

"Well, the funny thing about the goblet squat . . . is that it answers the question: What do the hips do? And if . . . the kettlebell 'reverse engineers' the action of the hips, . . . then in the goblet squat, the movement greases that key human motion: the squat." And so there you have it in plain speech, by Dan John himself, master strength coach and originator of the goblet squat.

The goblet squat is the speediest way to get someone squatting properly and quickly. Really, it's nearly impossible to do wrong. The following steps walk you through it:

1. **Grab a kettlebell or dumbbell and hold it directly in front of the chest, like a goblet (hence, the name *goblet squat;* see Figure 5-8a).**

   Keep the weight held as snuggly to the chest as possible.

2. **Assume a little wider than hip-width stance, and point your toes slightly out. This is your squatting stance.**

3. **Start the movement by sitting down, as if you're reaching your butt down for a curb. (It may help to think that you're pulling yourself down between your legs.)**

   Keep in mind that in a squat, you sit down; in a swing, you sit back.

4. **Continue to descend for as long as you're able to keep your heels on the ground, your knees in line with your toes, and your back flat (see Figure 5-8b).**

5. **When you stand up, be sure that your hips and shoulders ascend simultaneously.**

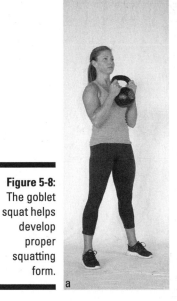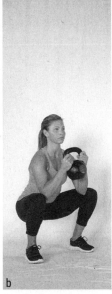

Figure 5-8: The goblet squat helps develop proper squatting form.

Photos courtesy of Rebekah Ulmer

The bodyweight squat

It may strike you as odd that we put the bodyweight squat after the goblet squat in terms of progressions, but we have our reasons. Mostly, we've done this because the bodyweight squat is horribly overworked, and people generally lack the authentic mobility and stability to properly do one.

So don't be surprised when you discover that the goblet squat comes easier than a bodyweight squat. The natural counterbalance of the weight helps compensate for mobility issues, allowing for a greater range of motion with better form.

With that being said, the bodyweight squat is still great, and it should be everyone's goal to perform one beautifully. Here's how:

1. **Assume a hip-width stance and point your toes slightly out.**

2. **Reach your arms out in front of you for balance (see Figure 5-9a) and begin to sit down, pulling yourself between your legs.**

   Your knees *will* come forward in a squat; just be sure they stay in line with your toes.

3. **Go as low as you can, keeping your heels on the ground, your knees in line with your toes, and your back flat (see Figure 5-9b).**

   Do your best to keep your weight evenly distributed throughout your feet.

4. **When you stand up, be sure your hips and shoulders ascend simultaneously.**

Figure 5-9: The challenge with the bodyweight squat is maintaining balance.

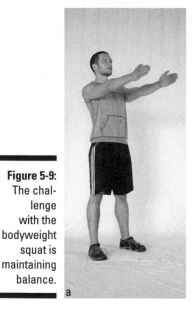 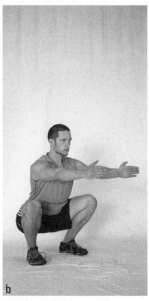

a   b

Photos courtesy of Rebekah Ulmer

The goblet lunge

The lunge isn't a squat per se, but it's still a knee, or quad, dominant movement, and it's still an extremely valuable one at that. The lunge is effectively a squat taken from a split stance, or more simply, a sort of single-leg squat. Because most of your movement occurs either from a split stance or as the result of pushing off just one leg, you want to train the unilateral (one-limb) movements, such as the lunge, just as extensively as you train the bilateral (two-limb) movements, such as the squat.

You can perform the lunge with either a weight held in the goblet position (like you would a goblet squat) or with no weight at all. You may find that holding a weight in front of your chest may assist with balance and posture. Follow these steps to do the goblet lunge:

1. **Assume a hip-width stance and hold the weight in front of your chest as you would a goblet squat (see previous section).**

2. **Begin by stepping back deeply with one leg (see Figure 5-10a), maintaining the hip-width stance. Imagine you're lunging on railroad tracks.**

   Maintain a fairly square and upright torso throughout the lunge. That means don't lean forward, twist, or rotate. Also don't go too narrow with your stance, unless you want to topple over.

3. **Continue to lunge back until the knee of your back leg reaches the ground (see Figure 5-10b). You may rest your knee there, but don't bang it.**

   Notice that in the lunge both feet are pointing forward.

4. **To come out of the lunge, push equally off your front leg and back leg and return to the starting position.**

   Be sure to keep your back toes tucked, not pointed, so you can push off the ball of your back foot when lunging.

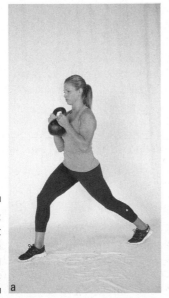
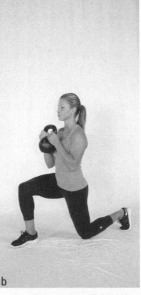

Figure 5-10: The goblet lunge is like a single-leg squat.

a   b

Photos courtesy of Rebekah Ulmer

Intermediate Squatting Exercises

After your squatting mechanics are sound, you can start to load the movement considerably. With squats, and with most movements relating to the squat, you can move a lot of weight, and sometimes, that's precisely what you should do.

When you load a movement — meaning you add weigh to it — you cement the pattern. Don't push the weight until your form is near faultless.

The two exercises in this section are our favorite variations for adding more weight to squats and lunges in the quickest and safest manner possible.

The racked squat

With a racked squat, you perform a squat with weight held in the rack position (in front of your chest). This squat is best done with two kettlebells, two dumbbells, or a sandbag. Racked squats stress the core in a unique way and light up your abs.

When starting out with "racked" exercises, start with just one weight (either a kettlebell or dumbbell) in the rack to get accustomed to the position before moving onto two weights.

Follow these steps to do a racked squat:

1. **Clean the weight up into the rack position (see the earlier section on the clean).**

   Keep your forearms vertical and tight against your rib cage (see Figure 5-11a). Take a small step if needed to assume your squatting stance (feet, shoulder-width apart; toes out).

2. **Take a deep breath into your belly and start your squat.**

   Imagine you're pulling yourself down between your legs. Keep your back flat, heels on the ground, and knees in line with the toes (see Figure 5-11b).

   Be sure to keep air in your belly throughout the movement to help keep your spine safe.

3. **When you've hit your maximum depth, push your heels into the ground, drive your hips forward, and stand up.**

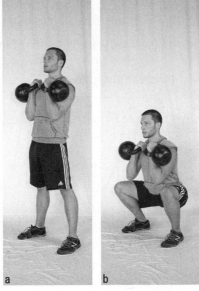

Figure 5-11:
A racked
squat
with two
weights.

a   b

Photos courtesy of Rebekah Ulmer

The racked lunge

The racked lunge not only lets you load more weight onto the movement, but it may also provide an additional challenge for your core — especially if you're using two different size weights. You'll know it when you feel it.

And, yes, you can use two different size weights for just about any exercise, and from time to time, we encourage you to do just that. Rarely in life do you pick up anything that's perfectly even in weight. So it doesn't need to be that way inside the gym either.

Here are the steps for the racked lunge:

1. **Clean the weight into the rack position and assume your squatting stance (see the earlier sections for these movements and Figure 5-12a).**

    Keep your stance approximately shoulder-width throughout the lunge to keep your balance.

2. **Step back into a deep lunge (see Figure 5-12b).**

   You may plant your hind knee on the ground; just don't bang it.

3. **Push hard from both your front and hind legs to stand up out of the lunge.**

   Be sure to keep your back toes planted (not pointed) so you can push off the ball of your foot (rather than your instep) when lunging.

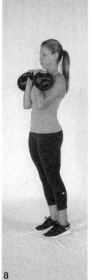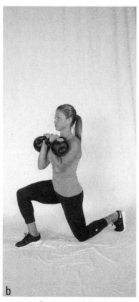

Figure 5-12:
A racked lunge with two weights.

a   b

Photos courtesy of Rebekah Ulmer

Advanced Squatting Exercises

In the advanced category, we discuss only two movements. The front squat allows you to move a considerably larger load through the squatting pattern than the intermediate racked or goblet squats. Due to the placement of the weight, it requires more shoulder mobility, too. The second exercise — the pistol squat — serves as one of the best single-leg bodyweight exercises in existence for strengthening the lower body.

The front squat

You want to perform the front squat with a barbell, solely for the reason that you can load more weight onto a barbell than you can handle with a set of kettlebells or dumbbells. But other than the amount of weight, and the placement of the weight, the movement pattern is identical to the goblet squat or racked squat (discussed earlier in this chapter) — so don't move too hastily onto the front squat until you have those two movements mastered.

Note: To perform the front squat, you also need a rack to hold the barbell in between sets.

Here's how to do the front squat:

1. **Set up under the barbell so it lies across the front of your shoulders just above your clavicle and close to your throat (see Figure 5-13a).**

   Hold the barbell with a *clean grip* — where your fingers loosely grip the bar just outside of your shoulders while you drive your elbows up and in until your forearms are parallel with the ground. Support the weight with your body, not your arms; the clean grip simply acts as a placeholder for the weight across the front of your shoulders.

2. **Stand up out of the rack, and step away.**

   Get in the habit of taking as few steps as you need to find your squatting stance — there's no point in wasting time or energy messing around with your stance.

3. **Take a deep breath into your belly and start your squat (refer to the earlier section "The goblet squat" for the basic squat form, and see Figure 13b).**

   As always, keep your back flat, heels on the ground, and knees in line with your toes.

   It's imperative to keep air in your belly when under load. Breathe out while pushing your tongue against the roof of your mouth when coming out of your squat (to maintain intra-abdominal compression), but just don't breathe all your air out.

4. **When you've hit your maximum depth, push your heels into the ground and drive your hips forward to stand up and finish the movement.**

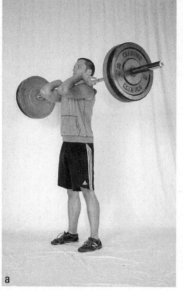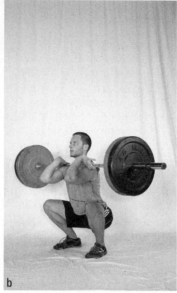

Figure 5-13: The front squat with a barbell.

a

b

Photos courtesy of Rebekah Ulmer

You're not done with the front squat until the barbell is placed safely back on the rack. Just because you have completed the rep doesn't mean you can relax. Stay tight and maintain good form the entire time you're under the bar.

The pistol squat

The pistol squat is a full squat on one leg. It sounds simple, but, as you probably know, simple isn't always easy — and the pistol squat is an undeniable testament to that fact.

The pistol squat requires not only brute strength but also stability, mobility, balance, and coordination. It's not only a fantastic leg strengthener in itself but also a viable metric of your overall movement abilities. If you can do a pistol squat, you have gained a lot; if you can't, you have a lot to gain.

You can do the pistol squat with or without weight. Often, people find the pistol squat is more accessible when they're allowed to hold a small weight out in front as a counterbalance. Experiment and see what works best for you. Follow these steps for the pistol squat:

1. **Assume a shoulder-width stance and extend your arms out in front as a counterbalance.**

   If you choose to weight the pistol squat, hold it in the goblet or rack position (see earlier sections for these positions).

2. **Lift one leg straight up off the ground (see Figure 5-14a); the higher you can get it up, the better.**

   Try to keep your elevated leg fully extended out in front of you throughout the entire movement. It may even help to keep your toes pointed straight up. Also, be sure to start with your working leg heel on the ground.

3. **Begin to squat down as low as you can on one leg (see Figure 5-14b) while keeping your heel on the ground, your knee in line with your toes, and your back as flat as possible.**

   If you keep falling on your butt, try holding a light weight out in front of you to act as a counterbalance, as shown in Figure 5-14b.

4. **When you hit rock bottom (if you're able), push your heel hard into the ground and drive your hips forward to stand up.**

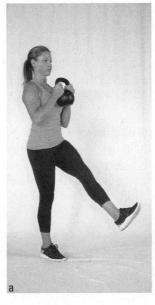
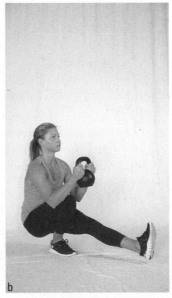

Figure 5-14: You do the pistol squat with one leg out in front of you.

a

b

Photos courtesy of Rebekah Ulmer

Hinging Skill Drills

Having trouble finding your hinge? No worries, the troubleshooting drills in this section will help you fix any movement bugs. And if you're trying to decide whether you need these drills, the answer is you do. Everyone does. No matter how well you move, you can always gain something from going back and reworking the basic fundamental movement patterns.

The broomstick drill

The broomstick drill shows you what a neutral spine should feel like. From the outside, a neutral spine should look like a relatively flat back — no excessive arching or rounding. The spine itself is still curved, but nothing should look overly pronounced.

To perform this drill, you need a broomstick or some other long, straight, and thin object that you can line up alongside your back. The purpose of this drill is to line three parts of your backside alongside the broomstick to force you into a neutral position. Here's how:

1. **Grab a broomstick (or something of the sort) and line it up on your back so that it touches three points of contact.**

   Make sure you find a broomstick long enough to reach from the top of your head down to your tailbone. The first point you want the broomstick to touch is the very back of your head, the second point is your upper back (your thoracic spine), and the third point is your tailbone (sacrum).

2. **Hold the broomstick with one arm behind your neck and one arm behind your low back (see Figure 5-15a). Don't overarch your lower back.**

3. **While maintaining these three points of contact on the broomstick, start to perform a few sets of hinges (see the earlier sections on hinges in this chapter and check out Figure 5-15b).**

If at any time the broomstick disengages from any of the three points, reset and try again. Pay extra attention to your tailbone, because many times that's the first point of contact to leave the stick.

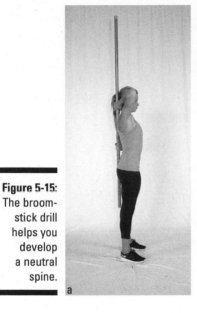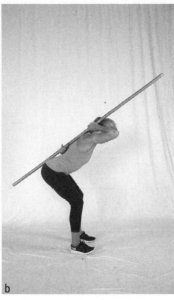

Figure 5-15:
The broom-stick drill helps you develop a neutral spine.

Photos courtesy of Rebekah Ulmer

The butt-to-wall drill

The butt-to-wall drill helps you find your optimal hinge position. In short, it shows you where exactly you should be sticking your butt. And all you need to do this drill is a chunk of wall.

1. **Find an unoccupied wall (or have someone hold a broomstick as shown in Figure 5-16a) and stand directly in front of it facing away.**

2. **Assume your hinging stance (see the earlier sections on hinges in this chapter), reach your butt back, and touch the wall (see Figure 5-16b).**

   Keep a straight line from the back of the head down through the tail-bone, as shown in Figure 5-16b.

3. **Take a small step forward, reach your butt back, and touch the wall again.**

4. **Continue to repeat Step 3 until you find the farthest possible point you can be away from the wall but still reach it with your butt. This is your optimal hinge position.**

   If you fall backward, you've gone too far. Step back toward the wall a little bit and try again.

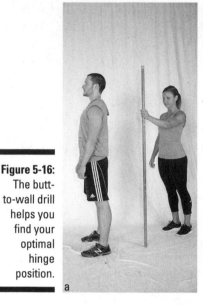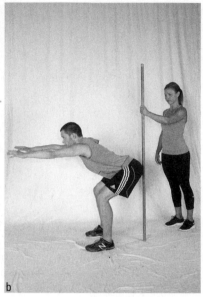

Figure 5-16:
The butt-
to-wall drill
helps you
find your
optimal
hinge
position.

a   b

Photos courtesy of Rebekah Ulmer

Squatting Skill Drills

The deep squat, if you don't already have it, can be a hard movement to regain. But if you practice these skill drills diligently — *diligently* being the most important word here — you can reclaim this movement. Don't expect to restore your squat overnight, over a couple days, or even over a couple weeks. Just be patient; it will come.

Primal pole dancing

The purpose of this drill is to find something to assist you into the deep squat position. You can use just about any object that's waist height or higher — a pole or a door are both perfectly suitable:

1. **Grab hold of the pole or door and use it to help wedge yourself down into a deep squat (see Figure 5-17).**

If someone is available, you may use a partner for this drill as well. Just have the person hold onto your hands to counterbalance you as you move into a deep squat.

2. **When you hit rock bottom, drive your knees and shins forward while keeping your heels glued to the ground.**

   This action will help mobilize what often restricts your squat — your ankles — but it only works if you keep your heels on the ground. Work this for as many repetitions as necessary.

3. **Spend as much time in the bottom of the squat position as you want.**

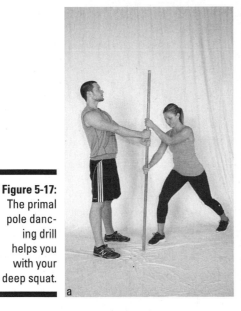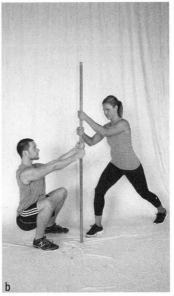

Figure 5-17: The primal pole dancing drill helps you with your deep squat.

a   b

Photos courtesy of Rebekah Ulmer

The frog stretch

The frog stretch unglues the hips and is a great way to mimic the squat without actually squatting. All you need to perform the frog stretch is a piece of ground. Follow these steps:

1. **Get down on your hands and knees, lining your hands under your shoulders and your knees under your hips.**

2. **Set your back flat if it isn't already and spread your knees out as wide as you possibly can (see Figure 5-18a).**

3. **Drop down onto your forearms and begin to drive your hips backward (see Figure 5-18b).**

   If you are having trouble with rounding your back, you may want to exaggerate the arch in your low back for this movement.

4. **Continue to drive the hips back until you start to feel the stretch; hold it, breathe, and try to relax into a deeper range of motion.**

   When stretching, the goal is to relax, not to force anything open. Spend as much time in the frog stretch as you need; the longer, the better.

5. **To come out of the stretch, slowly drive your hips forward and bring your knees back together.**

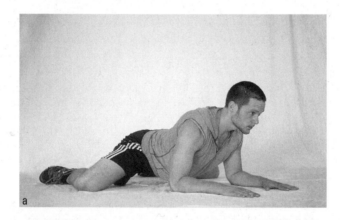

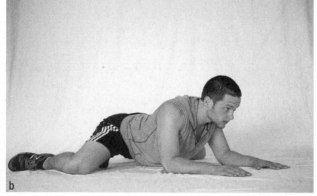

Figure 5-18:
The frog stretch helps you relax into a deeper range of motion.

Photos courtesy of Rebekah Ulmer

Chapter 6

Pushes and Pulls for a Stronger, Harder Torso

In This Chapter

▶ Developing a truly perfect push-up

▶ Working your way to your first pull-up — and beyond!

▶ Mastering proven progressions and skill drills

T he chapters in this part of the book are here to help you understand movement quality. We must warn you not to press forward into the primal fitness programs prematurely. You need to have dominance over the fundamental primal movements before you slam it into high gear. If you don't, then it's like you're driving with the emergency brake on and you'll progress slower than you would otherwise. Or even worse, you're driving with no brakes at all and are bound to injure yourself.

In this chapter, we move to upper body movements and cover the fundamental pushing and pulling exercises found within the primal exercise programs. If you're new to exercise, we show you how to do a *truly* perfect push-up and how to get your first pull-up. If you're a veteran, we challenge you with the one-arm push-up, the one-arm one-leg push-up, and the elusive one-arm chin-up.

The minor function of all these exercises, of course, is to develop raw upper body strength, inexhaustible power, and eye-catching aesthetics. The major function, and the one most overlooked, is to develop beautiful, functional movement.

All about the Primal Pushes

In the domain of pushes, we have two categories. The first is a horizontal push, such as the push-up. We classify this push as horizontal not because the push-up has you in a horizontal position but because if performed standing, the movement would be horizontal to the floor. The second is a vertical push, such as an overhead military press. Naturally, countless angles and variations exist between these two exercises.

If we haven't made it clear enough by now, all the movements in this book are big, full-body movements. We don't focus on "isolation" (or bodybuilding) training. We choose not to train muscle groups independently but rather collectively and synergistically, because this is how the body is meant to move.

In the body, everything is connected, and everything is meant to work together. Therefore, "isolation" training or single muscle group training is somewhat misleading. With Paleo fitness, we focus on the big, compound movements that work multiple muscle groups simultaneously. It's better that way.

Reaping the benefits of the big pushes

Upper body strength is just one of the benefits of pushes. And with that upper body strength, you achieve robust, durable shoulders. And how about a torso that's the envy of the neighborhood? Yes, you can most assuredly expect all of this and more from the movements throughout this chapter.

But there's more: When you make your way into the more advanced pushing variations, such as the infamous one-arm one-leg push-up, you quickly discover that these pushes develop much more than upper body strength. Perhaps, it'd be more appropriate to say that just about all these exercises are really full-body movements with an upper body emphasis. You see what we mean when you feel how the push-ups and overhead presses sneakily attack core and lower extremities as well.

And don't let the "advanced" stuff intimidate you. Again, Paleo fitness is about progressing at your own pace. No matter what level you're at, we give you a starting place where you'll be challenged but successful. And that is the key.

Practicing strength

People often think that strength is the result of bigger muscles. This idea is true in part — a relatively small part, that is. Strength is more neurological than anything else, meaning it stems first from the central nervous system. A useful and common analogy is to think of your muscles as the factory, your central nervous system as the manager, and strength as the output. To increase the output, you can do one of three things: (1) Increase the size of the factory (build bigger muscles); (2) increase the efficiency of the manager (train the nervous system); or (3) do a combination of both.

In other words, you don't have to be "big" to be strong. Many athletes, like gymnasts for example, display an almost superhuman level of strength, yet they don't sport the bulky frame of a bodybuilder. That's because these athletes have a very finely tuned nervous system. They're highly efficient machines and have become so by training their nervous system first, not by bulking their muscles.

We tell you this now because many of the movements in this chapter — such as the one-arm push-up — will, at first, feel very difficult. We want to assure you that with assiduous practice, they'll feel less and less difficult over time. Efficiency comes with practice.

If you want to get better at a particular movement, practice it as often as you can throughout the day. Try setting yourself a daily, or even an hourly, quota of reps. Keep the reps low, though, to avoid too much fatigue (when practicing an exercise, you want to feel as fresh as possible). For example, do you want to get better at pull-ups? Start by doing just one pull-up every hour you're awake. You'll be amazed how much stronger you feel at pull-ups even after one week!

Beginner Pushes

We're willing to bet you know exactly what exercise we introduce in this section. We're also willing to bet that you'll soon have a newfound appreciation and understanding of this classic exercise: the push-up.

Here, we show you the push-up and the military press — one horizontal push and one vertical push. Together, these two movements will help make you strong at just about every angle.

The push-up

Is the push-up the perfect primal exercise? In many ways, yes, it is. It hits hard not only the primary pushing muscle group — chest, triceps, and shoulders — but also many unsuspecting parts of the body, such as the abs. It can be easily scaled to accommodate all strength levels, and it's perhaps the most shoulder-friendly pushing exercise.

Unfortunately, many people discount the push-up because they feel it's too easy; they think there isn't as much to be gained with the push compared to lifting weights. They're wrong. You gain strength from working against resistance. Whether that resistance is your own body weight or external weight is irrelevant. Your muscles don't know the difference. Neither does your brain.

Yes, the push-up by itself can take you only so far, and if you can rep out 15 or so push-ups with faultless form, then it's likely time for you to move on to a more difficult variation, such as the one-arm push-up or the one-arm one-leg push-up. On the other hand, if you've had a difficult time achieving even just one push-up, don't worry: We show you how to get there in the following steps. And if you do what we say, it won't take you long, either.

1. **Set up in the top of a push-up position so your hands are directly under your shoulders and your feet are together (see Figure 6-1a).**

   The top of the push-up is identical to the top of a plank. Follow the "rule of thumb" — your thumb should be inside your shoulders when setting up for a push-up.

2. **Brace your abs and squeeze your butt.**

   This step often helps fix alignment issues. You should have a straight line from the back of your head all the way down through your tailbone.

3. **As you descend into the push-up, keep your elbows pointed back and tucked in to your sides (see Figure 6-1b).**

   A vertical forearm is a marker of a proper push-up form.

4. **When you hit rock bottom (elbows bent to at least 90 degrees), push hard into the ground and drive back up into a full lockout position (elbows fully extended).**

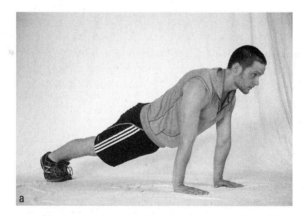

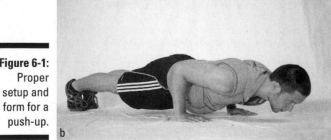

Figure 6-1:
Proper
setup and
form for a
push-up.

Photos courtesy of Rebekah Ulmer

If you have trouble performing a strict push-up, continue to work the push-up from your feet but do so on a slight incline. (We don't like push-ups from the knees because they encourage poor mechanics and rarely help build the strength required for a full push-up.) The easiest variation is to perform push-ups on a set of stairs so your hands are elevated. As you get stronger, lessen the incline, and continue to work your way down to the floor. See the "Pushing Skill Drills" section, later in this chapter.

Strength comes from practice. If you want to get good at push-ups, then you have to practice push-ups! The best way to practice is to perform a few push-ups intermittently throughout the day. You can even try setting yourself a daily, or hourly, push-up quota.

The military press

The military press is an old-timey strength builder, one that fell slightly out of fashion with the advent of the bench press but is slowly starting to come back. The military press is one of the most effective upper body grinding exercises found anywhere. It builds "real-world" overhead strength — some would call that "dad strength."

The military press toughens the shoulders and brutalizes the abs in a way the bench press can't. This movement is best performed with either one or two kettlebells or dumbbells or a barbell. We suggest you start out practicing this movement with a single kettlebell or dumbbell, and then work your way into double kettlebell/dumbbell and barbell pressing. All the same rules apply.

Here are the steps for the military press:

1. **Clean a kettlebell or dumbbell up into the rack position. (See Chapter 5 for steps to the clean and check out Figure 6-2a.)**

2. **Brace the abs, squeeze your butt, and take in a deep breath of air.**

3. **Begin to press the weight up overhead; try to keep your forearm vertical throughout the entire press (see Figure 6-2b).**

   Don't lean back during the military press. Keep the abs tight and the spine neutral!

4. **Press to a full lockout position, as shown in Figure 6-2c.**

   Your bicep should be in line with, or slightly behind, your ear at the top position.

5. **Pull the weight all the way back down to the rack position, and repeat.**

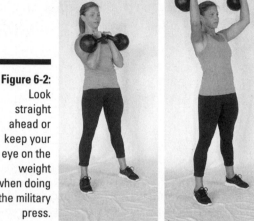

Figure 6-2:
Look
straight
ahead or
keep your
eye on the
weight
when doing
the military
press.

a   b   c

Photos courtesy of Rebekah Ulmer

Intermediate Pushes

The intermediate pushes are the bench press and the one-arm push-up. You should have a strong handle on both the push-up and the military press to prep the shoulders and assess their tolerance before moving on to the bench press. And the one-arm push-up simply isn't possible unless you already have a strong push-up foundation.

When you're ready for these exercises, they will blast you into previously undreamt of levels of upper body strength!

The one-arm push-up

The one-arm push-up develops strength in ways few exercises can. This movement requires total body control, intense focus, and raw strength. The one-arm push-up is much more than a party trick. This exercise has tremendous carry-over into all sports and activities.

The one-arm push-up will seem near impossible at first attempt, but don't give up. The progressions in the "Pushing Skill Drills" section, later in this chapter, will have you repping out one-arm push-ups in no time! Here are the steps:

1. **Set up at the top of your push-up position (refer to Figure 6-1a).**

   Be sure to set up with your hand as close to in line with your sternum (lower chest) as possible to ensure the shoulder is kept in good position throughout the push-up.

2. **Split your stance.**

   Kick your opposite leg out like a kickstand to assist with balance. The farther you kick out your opposite leg, the more assistance it will lend to the movement.

3. **Lift the non-working arm off the ground. You may want to place it on your hip for balance (see Figure 6-3a).**

4. **Begin to descend into your one-arm push-up, keeping your elbow in close to your side (see Figure 6-3b).**

   The most difficult part of the one-arm push-up is keeping everything as square as possible. Don't let your shoulders or hips rotate throughout the movement.

5. **When you hit rock bottom (see Figure 6-3c), drive back up, following the same path you took on the descent.**

Your hip may deviate outward a little bit when performing the one-arm push-up; just be sure to keep it to a little bit.

The bench press

No one can ignore the bench press or deny its effectiveness. Admittedly, this exercise isn't for everyone, but for those who have the shoulders for it, the bench press offers huge strength returns.

You may or may not have the shoulders to handle bench pressing. If you experience any pain or discomfort with this movement, stop immediately. You can also exchange push-up variations for bench pressing.

The bench press is best performed with a barbell because it allows you to load the most weight onto the movement. And really, the ability to move the most weight through the greatest range of motion is the major benefit of the bench press over the other pushing exercises. However, if you feel more comfortable bench pressing with dumbbells or kettlebells, go for it.

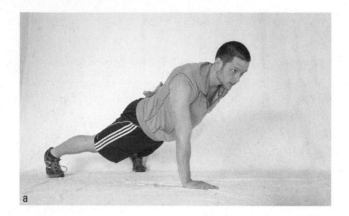

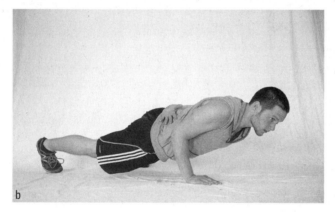

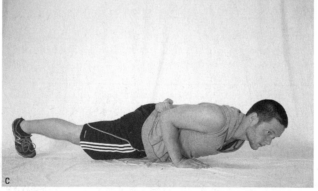

Figure 6-3:
A one-arm
push-up
is surely a
feat!

Photos courtesy of Rebekah Ulmer

Here's how to properly execute a bench press:

1. **Lie down on the bench, planting your feet on the ground.**

   Make sure the bench touches your butt and upper back at all times and maintain the natural curvature of your spine (neutral spine) throughout the movement.

2. **Grab the bar just outside of shoulder-width, maybe a little wider. Place the bar deep into the heel of your palm to take some stress off the wrist (see Figure 6-4a).**

   If you need to, use a spotter to help you lift the barbell up into the starting position. In fact, it's best to have a spotter at all times during the bench press.

   Don't go too wide with your grip, or you may irritate your shoulders.

3. **Keep your elbows within a 45-degree angle as you lower the bar down toward your sternum (see Figure 6-4b).**

   The forearms should be vertical or very close to vertical at the bottom of the bench press, as shown in Figure 6-4c. To help keep your shoulders in a good position and your elbows in the right spot, imagine that you're trying to bend that bar like a horseshoe throughout the bench.

4. **Drive the bar back up and over your face. The bar shouldn't travel straight up and down but rather in a C pattern.**

   Don't forget to breathe! Take a deep breath into the belly as you lower the bar, and let out a compressed breath as you press it back up. Also, be sure to press back up to a full lockout with each rep.

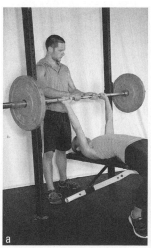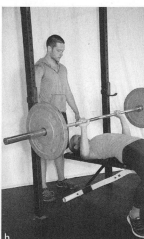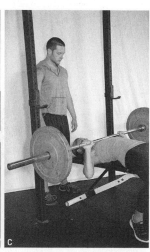

Figure 6-4: If you need to, use a spotter when doing the bench press.

Photos courtesy of Rebekah Ulmer

The dip

You can perform the dip on a set of parallel bars, gymnastic rings, or straps. We suggest you develop the dip first on the most stable surface: the parallel bars. After that, we prefer gymnastic rings because they make for the greatest challenge and allow for more freedom of movement.

The dip is most commonly seen in gymnastics training. It strengthens the shoulder and the elbow joints (just be careful not to push it too far or too much at first), while building the deltoids, chest, and triceps.

Here are the steps to the dip:

1. **Stabilize yourself on top of a set of parallel bars (or rings or straps). Lock your elbows and keep your body as close to vertical as possible (see Figure 6-5a).**

   Don't let your shoulders shrug up. Press yourself away from the bars/rings.

2. **Slowly start to bend your elbows and come down into the dip.**

   To lessen the stress on your shoulders, you may begin to lean slightly forward, tilting your body into a more horizontal position. Continue until your elbows reach a 90-degree bend (see Figure 6-5b).

3. **Press back up into a full lockout position.**

Figure 6-5:
Ease your way into the dip so your shoulders get accustomed to the movement.

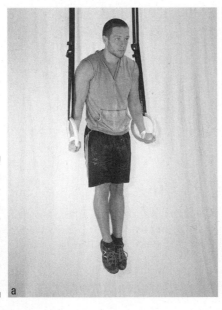 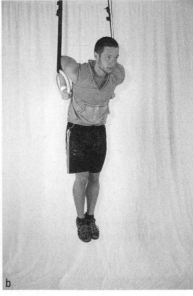

a b

Photos courtesy of Rebekah Ulmer

Advanced Pushes

The two exercises in this section use only body weight, but don't underestimate their difficulty. If you aim to conquer the one-arm one-leg push-up and the handstand push-up, you need to be patient with them.

When you master these two movements, you'll pretty much have all you'll ever need as far as upper body strength goes. Sure, there are greater feats to master, but we'd guess that just being able to do these two movements will by default place you in the top 1 percentile. And that's not too shabby.

The one-arm one-leg push-up

The one-arm one-leg push-up calls for more core control and grinding strength than the standard one-arm push-up (see earlier section). Not surprisingly, it develops more, too. Here's how to do it:

1. **Set up at the top of your push-up position and lift one arm and the opposite leg off the ground (see Figure 6-6a).**

   For example, if you lift your left arm, lift your right leg off the ground; if you lift your right arm, lift you left leg. Take time to stabilize yourself before moving on to the next step. You should also remain on the ball of your foot throughout the movement. Grip the ground forcefully with your fingers and toes (if you're barefoot) to help stabilize yourself.

2. **Begin to descend into the push-up position, keeping your shoulders and hips square (see Figure 6-6b).**

3. **When you hit the deck (Figure 6-6c), drive back up to the starting position.**

   Core control is vital. Keep a flat back and minimize all rotation throughout the movement. Not twisting or rotating is hard, but the less you do, the more effective the movement will be.

The handstand push-up

We show you how to perform a handstand push-up against a wall. But eventually, you should work up to performing the push-up from a free balancing handstand, which is by no accounts an easy feat!

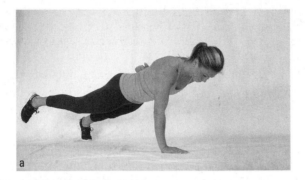

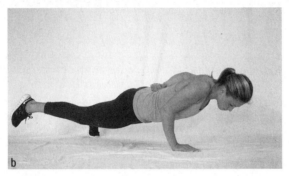

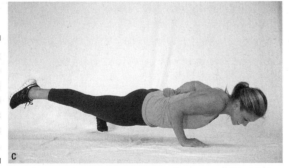

Figure 6-6:
The one-arm one-leg push-up requires tremendous control.

Photos courtesy of Rebekah Ulmer

Because you're inverted, this movement naturally falls into the vertical pushing category. It's more difficult than the standard push-up because you're moving a higher percentage of your body weight and you're doing so from a less advantaged position.

Here are the steps to the handstand push-up:

1. **Find a spot in front of the wall, and with your back toward the wall, place your hands on the floor shoulder-width apart fairly close to the wall. Keeping your elbows locked, kick your feet up so you're inverted and balanced against the wall.**

2. **Organize yourself in this inverted position. Shrug your shoulders up so they cover your ears, keep your belly tight (try to flatten out the arch in your back), put your legs together, and point your toes (see Figure 6-7a).**

   Spend as much as you need to get used to this position before attempting a push-up.

3. **Start to bend your elbows and lower yourself into the handstand push-up, moving your head closer to the ground, as shown in Figure 6-7b.**

   You want to get your head as close to the ground as possible, but don't bang it. Keep everything super tight and maintain the stiffness throughout your entire body. Don't force it. If something doesn't feel right, come out of the handstand.

4. **When your head reaches the floor, press back up into a full lockout to finish the movement.**

Figure 6-7:
Use a wall or a spotter to help you with the handstand push-up.

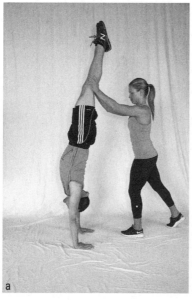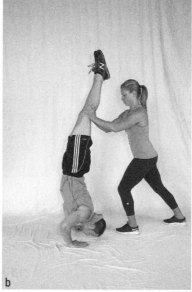

Photos courtesy of Rebekah Ulmer

All about the Primal Pulls

A push without a pull is as wrong as eggs without bacon. But because most people are after the "mirror muscles" — the pecs, the biceps, and the shoulders — they do way too much pushing and almost forget about pulling altogether. In fact, most people are so unbalanced, they would benefit from performing twice, or even three times, as many pulls as they do pushes!

In this section, we show you our favorite primal pulling movements to develop a strong, sinewy back and to balance out all that pushing!

Balancing out with pulls

Overemphasizing pushing and neglecting pulling eventually lead to some unwelcome imbalances, not to mention a weak back and poor posture. After you dive in to the primal fitness programs, you'll see that almost every push is balanced out with some sort of pull — either immediately or not too long after.

We admit that it'd be impossible to ever get the body perfectly balanced. But you should use exercise to correct imbalances, never to exaggerate them.

The easiest way to pair your pushes and pulls is to match the horizontal pushes with the horizontal pulls and the vertical pushes with the vertical pulls. For example, you can pair sets of push-ups with rows and sets of military presses with pull-ups. We provide more ways for you to balance out your routine in the workout programs in Part III, but for now, get into the habit of practicing pulls with all your pushes!

Recognizing the many benefits of pulling

Although nothing on it classifies as a "mirror muscle," a strong, muscular back is sure to grab the gaze of onlookers at the beach. A muscly posterior makes for a very aesthetically pleasing physique and a functional one, too!

Strengthening the musculature of the back — particularly the musculature that surrounds and supports the spine — improves your posture and invariably wards off back problems later on in life. Pulling naturally balances out the shoulders as well and helps to protect them from injuries brought on from imbalances.

And, yes, pulling makes you strong, too — very strong, if you follow the progressions in this book. We believe everyone (both male and female) should be able to pull their own body weight up to a bar for multiple repetitions.

Beginner Pulls

To build up your pulling strength, we start with rows and chin-ups. Don't worry if you don't have the chin-up down just yet; we give you a few variations to play with to help you along.

To work these exercises, you need something to hang from. For rows, a low bar or straps, such as a TRX suspension trainer, work nicely. For chin-ups, you need either a high bar, a set of gymnastic rings, or maybe even a tree branch.

The bodyweight row

The bodyweight row is a horizontal pulling exercise. You can think of it almost as a reverse push-up. The row strengthens just about all the muscles of the back as well as the shoulders and biceps.

Furthermore, the row is easily scaled, like the push-up, simply by adjusting your angle. For an easier row, start more upright. To increase the difficulty, work your way into a more horizontal position.

Here's how to do the bodyweight row:

1. **Grab hold of a bar or a set of straps.**

   If using straps, tug on them to make sure they're secure before leaning back.

2. **While holding on to the bar or straps, lean back and adjust your stance until you find a challenging angle to work from (see Figure 6-8a).**

   Be sure to keep your back flat, your shoulders back (don't let them pitch forward), and your armpits tight like you would in a swing. There should be a straight line running from the back of your head down through your tailbone, just as if you were in a push-up.

3. **Start to row yourself up by driving your elbows down toward your hips (see Figure 6-8b).**

   At the finish, your hands should land in line with your sternum.

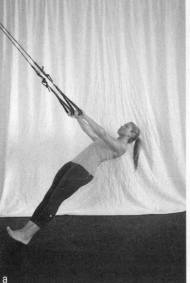 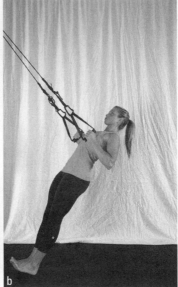

Figure 6-8:
In the bodyweight row, your body should move as one single unit — stiff as a board!

Photos courtesy of Rebekah Ulmer

The chin-up

The chin-up is a pull-up with your palms facing toward you. Because most people find the chin-up easier than a standard pull-up, it's a good place to start when working toward your first full pull-up.

The chin-up puts a greater emphasis on the biceps than the pull-up, which explains in part why some find the movement slightly easier. Nevertheless, it develops all the posterior pulling muscles and remains one of the most effective full-body strengthening exercises.

Here's how to do it:

1. **Grab hold of a bar with your hands shoulder-width apart and palms facing you. When your grip is secure, assume a dead hang (see Figure 6-9a).**

2. **Start the chin-up by sucking your shoulders down (think opposite of a shrug), bracing your abs, squeezing your butt (try to flatten the arch out of your back), and driving your elbows down hard toward your sides (see Figure 6-9b).**

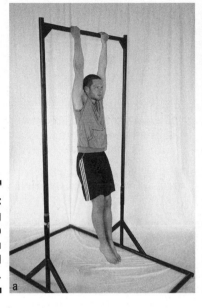 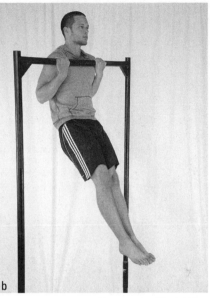

Figure 6-9:
Mastering
the chin-up
helps you
work toward
the pull-up.

a   b

Photos courtesy of Rebekah Ulmer

3. **Keep pulling until your throat reaches the bar — if you can get higher, great!**

   Don't try to complete a rep by reaching up with your chin. You either got it, or you don't; you won't get any stronger trying to fake it.

4. **Pause momentarily at the top, and then control yourself back down to a full dead hang before starting the next rep.**

Intermediate Pulls

After you master the beginner pulls, it's time to move on to some more challenging variations: the one-arm row and the pull-up. The one-arm row, just like the one-arm push-up (see earlier section), is difficult because it adds in an additional core challenge (rotation stability) and limits the effort to only one arm! And the pull-up, a classic test of upper body strength, is the next logical step after the chin-up.

Take your time and work toward these intermediate pulls only after you feel like you have a very strong foundation with the beginner pulls. Attempting to progress too soon will result in delayed progress.

The one-arm row

The one-arm row, quite simply, is the bodyweight row performed with one arm. Expect many of the same challenges with the one-arm row that you would with the one-arm push-up.

1. **Set up precisely how you would for a two-arm row (the more narrow your stance, the more difficult this movement will be; see earlier section "The bodyweight row"). Release one arm from the bar or straps, but keep your shoulders and your hips square (see Figure 6-10a).**

   The biggest challenge with this movement is fighting the rotation. Adjust your stance until you find a position where you'll be challenged but successful.

2. **Row yourself up with one arm. Your fist should finish in line with your sternum (see Figure 6-10b).**

   The difficulty of this movement also depends on the angle of your body in relation to the floor: More upright = less difficult; more horizontal = more difficult. Keep your shoulder pulled down and back by tensing your "armpit muscles"; don't allow it to be yanked forward.

3. **Control yourself back down to the starting position and repeat.**

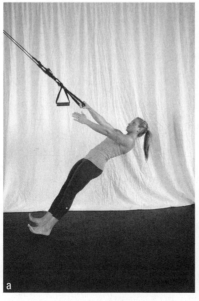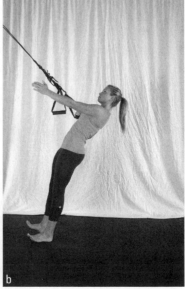

Figure 6-10:
The one-arm row using straps.

Photos courtesy of Rebekah Ulmer

The pull-up

Everyone should be able to do pull-ups, with very few exceptions. The pull-up is by all accounts one of the best back and upper body strengthening exercises. It is an exercise of the ages, if there ever was such a thing.

The pull-up punishes those with excessive body fat, and, interestingly enough, it may even be used as a sort of body fat analysis tool. For cxample, if you gain weight and your number of pull-ups stays the same, chances are the weight you've gained is muscle. But if you gain weight and your pull-ups go down, well, you've likely gained fat. The reverse also holds true when you lose weight.

If you can't do a pull-up, make it a priority and be diligent in your pursuit. We show you how to get there; you just have to put in the legwork — or armwork.

1. **Take a shoulder-width grip on the bar and assume a full dead hang position (see Figure 6-11a).**

2. **Initiate the pull-up by sucking your shoulders down, bracing your abs, squeezing your butt (try to flatten the arch out of your back), and driving your elbows down hard to your sides (see Figure 6-11b).**

   You may find it easier to engage your back if you imagine you're trying to "rip the bar apart" or "bend the bar in half" (like the bench press) while performing a pull-up.

3. **Continue to pull until your throat is against the bar, as shown in Figure 6-11c.**

4. **Control back down to a full dead hang position and repeat.**

   Don't just drop back into a dead hang because you may injure yourself. Control the descent.

Pull-ups make for a great exercise to practice intermittently throughout the day. Hang an easily removable pull-up bar, such as the Iron Gym brand, in your bathroom door. Every time you go to the bathroom, do five pull-ups.

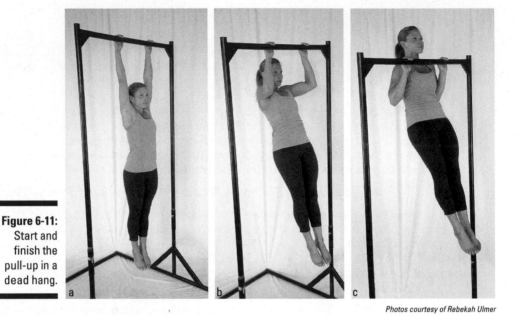

Figure 6-11: Start and finish the pull-up in a dead hang.

Advanced Pulls

The exercises in this section are heinous, plain and simple. To get to this level, you need raw strength, total body control, and technical proficiency. Oh, and a lot of patience, too. These movements sometimes take years to develop. If you think you're going to get to this point overnight, you're in for a disappointing morning.

The L-sit pull-up/chin-up is a fantastic exercise for the front and the backside. The muscle-up really combines pulling and pushing; it's essentially a pull-up into a dip. And the one-arm chin-up is very close to a circus act. All these exercises build tremendous strength.

The L-sit pull-up/chin-up

The L-sit will make a return in Chapter 7. We suggest you spend time practicing the L-sit by itself before working it in with your pull-ups or chin-ups. So if you're unfamiliar with the L-sit, you may want to jump to Chapter 7 to get the lowdown before proceeding here.

The L-sit turns a chin-up or a pull-up into a brutalizing core exercise. The entire body must maintain an adequate amount of tension; otherwise, the L-sit won't hold. This movement requires a strong set of abs and a strong back; it's surely one of the finest full-body movements anywhere.

Here are the steps for the L-sit pull-up/chin-up:

1. **Assume a pull-up or chin-up position (see the earlier sections on these exercises).**

2. **Raise your legs up to 90 degrees so your body forms an *L*. Lock your knees and point your toes (see Figure 6-12a).**

3. **While holding the L-sit, perform a full chin-up/pull-up (see Figure 6-12b).**

   To gain control and to increase its effectiveness, work this movement slowly.

Figure 6-12:
You must keep the abs under constant tension during the L-sit chin-up/pull-up.

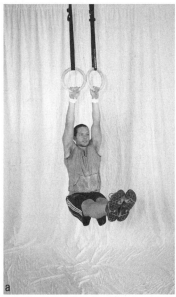 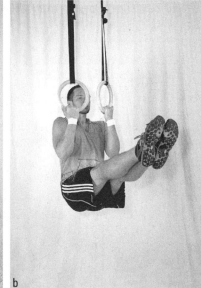

Photos courtesy of Rebekah Ulmer

The muscle-up

The muscle-up is a movement that comes from gymnastics and is best performed on a set of gymnastic rings. However, if you have only a bar to work with, you may use that instead.

The muscle-up is a pull-up into a dip. The most difficult part of this movement is the transition between the pull-up and the dip, where your elbows go from pointing down to pointing up. This transition requires strength through a range of motion that few people train.

The best ways to develop the strength for the muscle-up is to first get really strong at pull-ups and dips, and then begin working the muscle-up slowly in reverse. Nobody's first muscle-up is ever pretty. Just keep practicing.

The muscle-up can be quite stressful on unconditioned elbows and shoulders, so don't do too much too quickly. Your joints need time to toughen up.

Here are the steps for the muscle-up:

1. **Set up on the rings with a false grip (where the wrists are positioned over the rings, and the rings cut a diagonal across the bottom of the palm; see Figure 6-13a).**

   Developing the strength to hold a false grip takes a while. The best way to develop this strength is to start hanging with a false grip and practice pull-ups with a false grip as much as possible.

2. **Initiate a forceful pull-up, driving the rings down hard toward your sternum (see Figure 6-13b).**

   Imagine that you're trying to pull the rings through your sternum. Starting out, it may help to lean slightly back (almost like you would with a row) during the pull-up portion. Also, be sure to accelerate through the entire movement to avoid getting "stuck."

3. **After you've gained enough height, push your chest through the rings and pop your elbows up so you land in the bottom of a dip position (see Figure 6-13c).**

4. **Finish the movement by locking out the dip (see Figure 6-13d).**

   A full lockout on the muscle-up means your elbows are extended fully and shoulders are shrugged down.

The one-arm chin-up

The one-arm chin-up is a feat very few achieve. It's perhaps the ultimate test of upper body pulling strength. There are no tricks to the one-arm chin-up; it's a product of hard work and practice. If you want it, you have to work for it. Here are the steps:

1. **Assume a dead hang position from one arm from a bar or a set of rings. Keep the shoulders sucked down.**

   As you can see in Figure 6-14a, your body will naturally rotate sideways after you release one arm from the bar/ring.

2. **Tighten everything up like you would with a normal chin-up (see earlier section), drive your elbow down hard, and pull yourself up until your throat reaches the bar or rings (see Figure 6-14b).**

3. **Control back down to a full dead hang and repeat.**

Figure 6-13:
The most difficult part of the muscle-up is the transition.

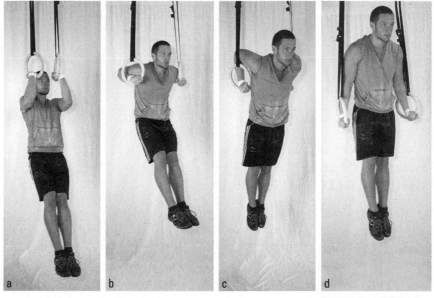

a   b   c   d

Photos courtesy of Rebekah Ulmer

Ease yourself into the one-arm chin-up practice. Elbow tendonitis is common with this movement from overuse.

One way to start developing the strength for the one-arm chin-up is to practice holding positions throughout the movement for time. For example, practice holding just the top position for a few seconds, then the middle, and everywhere in between.

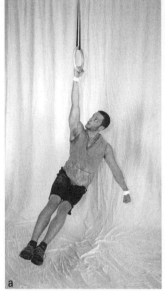 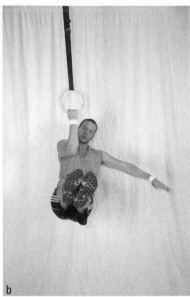

Figure 6-14:
The one-arm chin-up is the ultimate upper body pull.

a

b

Photos courtesy of Rebekah Ulmer

Pushing Skill Drills

In this section, we show you drills to refine your push-up technique and to progress toward the more advanced push-up variations. You can practice these drills separately on their own or work them into the primal fitness programs we outline in Part III.

The perfect push-up drill

The perfect push-up drill is a foolproof way to set up for, well, a perfect push-up! Here's how:

1. **Lie flat on your belly with your arms extended fully next to your sides (see Figure 6-15a).**

   Setting up the push-up from the bottom position helps ensure proper alignment.

2. **Reach your arms up behind you as high as you can, as shown in Figure 6-15b.**

   The higher you can lift your arms back up behind you in this position, the easier it will be for you to get your hands set up in the right spot.

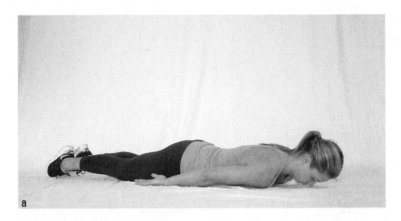

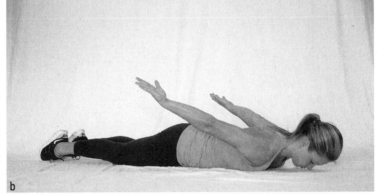

Figure 6-15:
Setting up for the perfect push-up.

Photos courtesy of Rebekah Ulmer

3. **Bend your elbows 90 degrees so your hands fall in line with your sternum (lower chest: see Figure 6-16a).**

   A perfectly vertical forearm is a marker of proper push-up form.

4. **Tuck your toes, tighten everything up, and set your back flat (so a straight line runs from the back of your head down through your tailbone throughout the entire push-up; see Figure 6-16b).**

   As you tighten up, lift slightly off the ground.

5. **Push up off the ground into a full lockout, ensuring that the shoulders, back, and hips all rise at the same time (see Figure 6-16c).**

   Keep your elbows tucked in close to your sides.

6. **Lower yourself back down to at least a 90-degree bend in your elbows and repeat.**

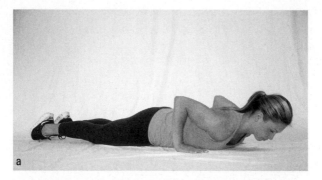

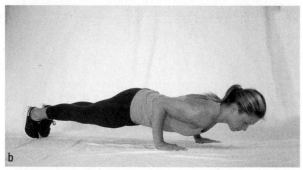

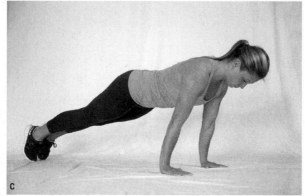

Figure 6-16:
Executing
a perfect
push-up.

Photos courtesy of Rebekah Ulmer

Finding your angle

One of the best push-up progressions, either for the standard push-up or any of the one-arm push-up variations, is to start working on a slight incline, such as a wall or a flight of stairs. When you develop proficient strength at that angle, begin to seek out objects that are a bit lower to the ground, such as a bench or a small box (see Figure 6-17). As you get stronger, continue to decrease the angle until you're performing your push-up (or push-up variation) on the ground.

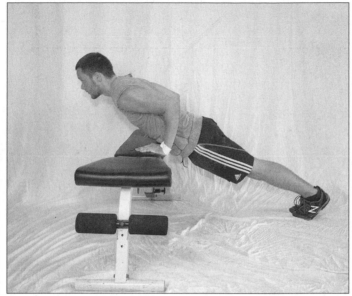

Figure 6-17:
Training on an angle is a great way to progress toward the more difficult push-up variations.

Photo courtesy of Rebekah Ulmer

Pulling Skill Drills

The pulling skill drills are geared toward helping you achieve your first pull-up. If you already have your first pull-up down, great; you can use the same ideas to progress toward the more difficult pulling variations.

The first pull-up is always the hardest to get, so be sure to set reasonable expectations for yourself. If you've never been able to do a full pull-up, then it's going to take a while — maybe even a couple of months. We remind you of this often, because it's easy to get discouraged when you don't see gains right away. But do what we say, keep practicing, and we promise you'll get there.

Flexed arm hangs

Flexed arm hangs are static positions — meaning "not moving" — held on a pull-up bar. Have someone, or something, assist you to the top of a pull-up bar and practice holding the top position, as shown in Figure 6-18. When you're able to hold the top position for a couple of seconds, practice holding as many other positions as possible throughout the pull-up.

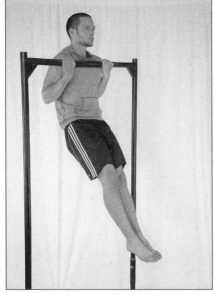

Figure 6-18:
Flexed arm hangs help you get used to holding up your own body weight.

Photo courtesy of Rebekah Ulmer

Negative pull-ups

Negative or eccentric pull-ups involve working only the downward portion of the pull-up (or chin-up). Have someone, or something, assist you to the top of a pull-up position. Then slowly control yourself all the way down into a dead hang position. The slower you can go, the better.

Chapter 7

Carrying Heavy Things and Ab Exercises That Don't Suck

· ·

In This Chapter

▶ Carrying heavy things without hurting yourself

▶ Strengthening the grip, shoulders, forearms, and torso

▶ Mastering functional core training

▶ Developing indestructible abs

· ·

arrying is perhaps the most primitive exercise of all and also perhaps the least performed in the gym. However, you see carrying regularly in many other occasions: the grocery store, the laundromat, or the playground. When people carry, they rarely do it with any true purpose or intent. It's simply the transportation of an object from one location to another through the means of human locomotion (that's movement).

Can you think of a more functional movement than carrying? We can't. People carry in some form every day without exception. Many of the other movements in this book, as marvelous as they are, are avoidable. Not every day demands a push-up, a pull-up, or a squat, but carrying is nearly inevitable, and we explore different types of carries in this chapter.

The cave man surely carried many heavy things and carried them quite often. We refer to carrying heavy things as *loaded carries,* a term coined by strength and conditioning coach Dan John. Loaded carries train everything all at once — the shoulders, the core, the legs. That's the simplest way to look at them at least. The loaded carry has jurisdiction over all the major muscle groups and punishes them all equally.

In this chapter, we also show you our prime selection of movements to strengthen, harden, and slenderize the midsection — what we refer to as "ab exercises that don't suck." We show you how to train your core in a functional manner — one that's in line with the core's true purpose — and ultimately how to carve out abs that will have you looking for opportunities to take you shirt off.

Mastering the Art of the Loaded Carry

Carrying is far from a fine art. It's an art of the simplest nature, really, kind of like finger painting. Out of all the movements in this book, loaded carries are probably the quickest skill to acquire. In fact, they're very hard to do wrong, but don't think this makes them easy. Although the skill is low, the effort often climbs to a very high altitude.

How a movement looks and how it feels are often two different things. Just because a movement or an exercise looks easy doesn't mean it will be easy to perform. Often, the very fine nuances are imperceptible to the untrained eye. A gymnast makes his routine on the rings look easy, but it'd be foolish to assume anything about the movements of a high-level gymnast are easy to perform.

In the following sections, we explore the art of carrying things, from fine-tuning everyday activities to developing strength and fitness with heavy loads.

Improving on an everyday activity

Try to get through a day without carrying something. If you're an able-bodied individual, not carrying *something* at some point in the day would be a difficult task. Whether it's a baby, a bag of groceries, or a backpack, people carry on almost all occasions, so you may as well do it right.

Every now and then you run into the mom (or dad) who tells the story of how carrying her baby — for all those *very long years* — ruined her back. Well, we're here to clear the baby's name. The truth is that the baby was never at fault for any back injury or pain. In fact, it's very unlikely that any baby ever had any intentions of purposefully wrecking its parent's back. It wasn't the carrying of the baby that led to back problems; it was *how* the parent carried the baby.

Lifting doesn't cause injury; how you lift causes injury.

Carrying heavy things for strength and fitness

Loaded carries strengthen the grip, improve posture, and peel away body fat. You can perform loaded carries anywhere and with just about anything. And we do mean anything — dumbbells, kettlebells, sandbags, logs, boulders, or even a small child, so long as the tyke is permitting.

The carryover from loaded carries into real life is likely higher than that of any other exercise found in this book and is as equally beneficial to the layperson as it is to the elite athlete. Loaded carries show you how to safely lift and transport heavy objects. If you've ever thrown your back out or tweaked this or strained that from lifting furniture, luggage, or whatever, then you can immediately see why carrying is a valuable skill to master.

From here on out, be conscious of how you lift and carry things. Whether it be as light as a notebook or as heavy as a couch, you should get into the habit of lifting and carrying it all in the same manner — with good form and proper body alignment. This is how you develop the habit of a safe lifting and carrying technique.

Beginner Carries

The two movements in this section, the farmer's carry and the waiter's carry, are as basic as it gets. But remember: You don't become elite because you move beyond the basics; you become elite when you move deeper into the basic movements — when you master them, perfect them, and own them.

No matter how strong you are now or will be, you'll never move beyond the basics. Yes, you'll begin to practice more "advanced" movements, but the basics will always be there, and you should continuously rehearse them, because the more you practice something, the more it becomes second nature.

Strength is a skill, and a skill is a habit of operation. If you want to be strong, move well, and perform optimally, you must get into the habit of rehearsing and strengthening your movement patterns with the utmost meticulousness — no matter how "basic" or "simple" they appear to be.

The farmer's carry

The farmer's carry is a classic strongman type of exercise. It's evident where the name comes from; what's not evident, however, is just how comprehensive this seemingly modest exercise is.

The famer's carry is one of the finest exercises for strengthening the grip and forearms. If Popeye had a favorite exercise, we'd guess the farmer's carry had to be it. The farmer's carry also reinforces good posture and core stability.

The famer's carry is most easily performed with a set of dumbbells or kettlebells, but really, you can perform it with just about anything you can hold on to — try a pail of water or a few buckets of sand if you really want to pay homage to the movement.

Here's how to do the farmer's carry:

1. **Dead lift one or two weights off the ground so they hang down by your sides. (See Chapter 4 if necessary to review proper dead lift technique.)**

   To set up for this exercise, set the weights up for the dead lift so they're outside of your feet, as shown in Figure 7-1a. This way, when you lift them up, they're right where you need them.

2. **Stand as tall as you can (imagine that you're trying to balance a set of books on your head), keep your shoulders "on the shelf" (that is, keep them back and don't let them hunch forward), and your core engaged (see Figure 7-1b).**

Figure 7-1:
Focus on good posture and a flat back for the farmer's carry.

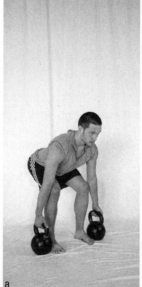
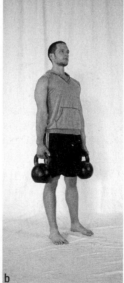

a   b

Photos courtesy of Rebekah Ulmer

The only way you can do this exercise wrong is to execute it with poor posture. Don't slouch or lean backward; stand as upright as possible. Think "long, tall spine" while you're holding the weight.

3. **Start walking, keeping your steps relatively small.**

   When you feel like you can't hold on with good form any more, set the weights back down just how you picked them up.

The waiter's carry

The waiter's carry is an overhead carry. This type of carry is slightly more demanding than the farmer's carry because it requires additional shoulder strength and mobility and core stability. Don't expect to be able to do this carry with as much weight as the farmer's carry; it just isn't going to happen.

The waiter's carry strengthens the shoulders in a very unique way, and aside from the Turkish get-up (see Chapter 3), it's one of the best ways to make your shoulders indestructible. This carry is best performed with either a kettlebell or a dumbbell. The following steps walk you through the waiter's carry.

If you can't achieve a full, stable lockout, don't do this movement. Simply perform the farmer's carry in its place until your shoulder mobility and stability improves.

1. **Clean a weight up (see Chapter 4 for details on the clean) into the rack position, press it overhead, and hold it there (see Figure 7-2a).**

   Take a few seconds to make sure everything feels okay before you start walking. Your elbow should be locked and your bicep should be next to your ear. Keep everything in line to support the weight. There should be a straight line down from the bell to the floor.

2. **Slowly start to walk around (see Figure 7-2b).**

   For an additional challenge, try walking on a slightly uneven surface outdoors.

Don't take any chances when you're holding weight overhead. If you don't feel like you can keep the weight up there or if something feels wrong, don't force it! Set the weight down, rest, and continue only when you feel confident.

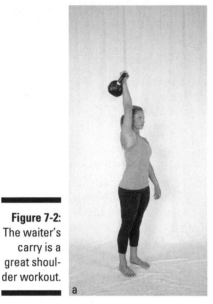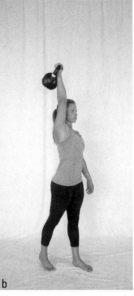

Figure 7-2:
The waiter's carry is a great shoulder workout.

a   b

Photos courtesy of Rebekah Ulmer

Intermediate Carries

In this section, we start to increase the load by moving from one-arm carries to two-arm carries. As you may expect, all the effects of the beginner carries will now be amplified. But don't rush into these intermediate carries too quickly; spend plenty of time building your foundation with the farmer's carry and waiter's carry in the previous section before venturing into the racked carry and two-arm waiter's carry.

The racked carry

The racked carry, and even just the rack hold for that matter, is one of the most boring-looking exercises but at the same time one of the most intense. Anyone who's spent time holding a considerable amount of weight in the rack position will quickly describe it to you as the direct opposite of a comfortable feeling, like an ever constricting straight jacket.

The racked carry presents a colossal total body stability challenge. The primary aim is to maintain poise and posture under the weight. That's it. The end result is a hardened and nearly unmovable frame, with the added benefit of an impervious set of abs.

The racked carry is best performed with two kettlebells. If you don't have a set of kettlebells, you can use dumbbells.

Follow these steps for the racked carry:

1. **Clean two kettlebells up into the rack position (see Chapter 5 for details). Be sure to keep everything as tight as you possibly can — bracing your abs, squeezing your glutes, and engaging your quads — and stand tall (see Figure 7-3a).**

   Don't lean back while you're in the rack position because doing so will immediately compromise your back. If at any time you catch yourself leaning back, set the weights down immediately.

2. **When you've gained a stable position, start to walk around in any direction you want (see Figure 7-3b).**

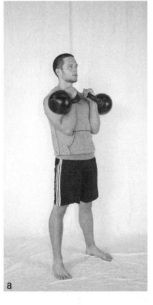 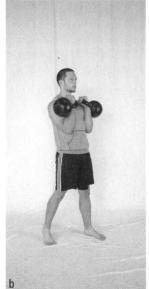

Figure 7-3: Maintain pose and posture in the racked carry.

a   b

Photos courtesy of Rebekah Ulmer

 When performing rack holds and racked carries, breathe shallow and into your belly. When the weight gets heavy, you'll find it nearly impossible to take a deep breath anyhow, so taking shallow breaths in this manner will help you keep your back safe and control the stress level.

The two-arm waiter's carry

Walking while holding weight overhead, especially two weights — two heavy weights — is an immense challenge. Everything in the body must be working together to make this happen. The core needs to be engaged, the shoulders need to be alert, and the legs need to be limber. All muscles are put to work in this movement.

Don't even think about trying this movement until you feel super confident with the regular waiter's carry (see earlier section). Supporting weight overhead yields a high return, but don't assume any more risk with this movement than necessary. Take your time and gain stability through the one-arm version first.

Here's how to do the two-arm waiter's carry:

1. **Clean two weights up to the rack position, press them overhead, and hold (see Chapter 5 for details on the clean, and check out Figure 7-4a).**

   Make sure all your body parts are neatly stacked. Make sure you aren't overarching your back or flaring out your rib cage; squeeze the abs and keep everything in proper alignment.

2. **When you feel ready, begin to slowly walk around in small steps (see Figure 7-4b).**

Figure 7-4:
In the two-arm waiter's carry, keep your forearms as close to vertical as possible.

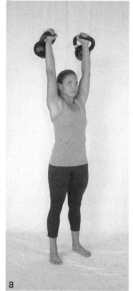
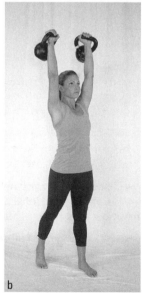

a   b

Photos courtesy of Rebekah Ulmer

Always err on the side of caution with overhead holds. Push yourself to a comfortable challenge but never into too much fatigue. Never let form deteriorate.

Advanced Carries: The Bottoms-Up Carry

The advanced carries — or *carry* — is of a different sort entirely. It isn't necessarily more difficult than the perspective of loading or mobility. What makes this movement "advanced" is the high degree of concentration and tension that you must maintain throughout. Also, the bottoms-up carry pulls a balancing component into the mix.

The bottoms-up carry can really only be performed with a kettlebell because it's one of the very few weight-training devices with an offset center of gravity. The bottoms-up carry, as the name implies, involves carrying the kettlebell in an inverted position — that is, with the handle below the actual weight. As you may expect, this position presents a colossal challenge for the grip, the abs, and the shoulders.

Don't expect to walk with this position at first. It will take you some time to be able to "catch" the kettlebell in the bottoms-up position from the clean and hold it there. It will take you double the time to get the hang of it on your non-dominant side.

Be sure to work with a kettlebell that's heavy enough; it must be a challenge to hold it in the bottoms-up position. If you choose too light of a weight, this profitable task becomes a joke.

Here's how to do the bottoms-up carry:

1. **Start to clean a kettlebell but, as the kettlebell begins to roll over onto your forearm, stop it halfway and hold it in the bottoms-up position (with the bottom of the kettlebell facing up toward the ceiling; see Figure 7-5).**

    To maintain the bottoms-up position, you have to squeeze everything — your abs, your butt, and, of course, the handle of the kettlebell!

2. **Stabilize your position. Keep your forearm perfectly vertical (otherwise, the bell will topple), and let the handle of the bell rest deep in the base of your palm.**

3. **When you've owned the position standing, start walking with it.**

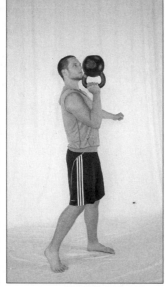

Figure 7-5:
The
bottoms-
up carry
requires
strength,
balance,
and coordi-
nation.

Photo courtesy of Rebekah Ulmer

To get better at the bottoms-up carry, you may want to start by practicing bottoms-up cleans for a while. The bottoms-up clean is simply performing a clean (see Chapter 5) but catching the kettlebell in the inverted or "bottoms-up" position rather than the rack position.

Getting the Abs of Your Dreams

Here we are at last. The section everyone has been waiting for. Just about everyone, at one time or another, has longed for a sleek, sexy set of abs.

Nothing is wrong with wanting six-pack abs. Just know that there are many ways to go about forging an indestructible midsection, some of them healthy, some of them not so healthy; some of them effective, and others not so effective.

Six-pack abs aren't always a reflection of good health. People often use extremely unhealthy methods to reduce body fat to a nearly nonexistent percentile. But with Paleo fitness, we take the opposite approach and guarantee your six-pack abs to be the result of vibrant health.

We're here to instruct you on how to perform the highest yield ab exercises on the planet. We're talking about functional core training that offers the highest return on your time and effort.

Functional training is a term that gets thrown around loosely and often without any true meaning. For us, functional core training must address the three primary functions of the core. The first of which is stability — that is, to maintain spinal position in the presence of change. The second is flexion and extension (think bend and unbend). The third involves rotation. The movements in the following sections cover all three.

Beginner Ab Exercises

In this section, we introduce two exercises: the four-point plank, which is a developer of core stability and a clear demonstration thereof, and the V-up, which is our preferred alternative to the classic crunch or sit-up. The V-up punishes the abs and teaches valuable alignment drills that you don't get with the crunch or the sit-up.

The four-point plank

Most likely, you're familiar with the plank. If not, think of the plank as the top of the push-up position (see Chapter 6). The name is symbolic of the looked-for body position, which should be flat; the hips shouldn't sag or pike up and neither should the belly.

The plank helps to develop linear core stability, or the ability to resist extension of the spine, which is the major function of your abs.

Here's how to do a perfect plank:

1. **Set up at the top of a push-up position; place your feet together and your hands directly under your shoulders (see Figure 7-6).**

   Keep your back flat at all times — no rounding or overarching — and keep everything in line, from head to tailbone.

2. **Hold the plank position for at least 20 seconds.**

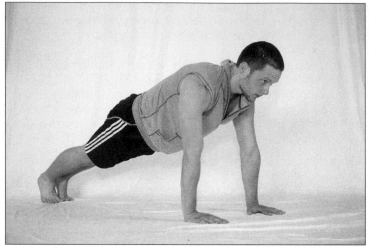

Photo courtesy of Rebekah Ulmer

3. **To get even more out of the plank, throw in some isometric contractions: Simultaneously squeeze your butt, abs, quads, triceps — every possible muscle that you can.**

   Adding in these contractions not only makes the plank more challenging but also serves to keep your body parts properly and neatly ordered.

The V-up

The V-up is a wonderful ab exercise to strengthen the abdominal wall, and it's typically much easier on the back than traditional sit-ups (which often aggravate or initiate back issues). The V-up is a useful progression toward the more challenging ab exercises, such as the hanging leg raise, which we introduce later in this chapter.

Perform the V-up on a relatively soft surface and follow these steps:

1. **Lie down flat on your back with your legs fully extended and your arms next to your side.**

2. **Squeeze your abs as hard as you can, trying to take the arch out of your low back (imagine you're trying to push your low back hard into the ground).**

This step results in what's often referred to as a *hollow position,* which looks sort of like a human banana. It's an excellent ab exercise by itself. Be sure to own this position before progressing forward.

3. **Slowly begin to raise your legs and torso simultaneously, trying to fold yourself in half while balancing on your buttocks (see Figure 7-7a).**

   Keep your legs straight the entire time. Go slowly; it will take some time before you're able to maintain your balance. You may rest your hands on the ground for balance when starting out, but eventually the goal is to perform this step without any "kickstands."

   For a more challenging variation, extend your arms up overhead, as shown in Figure 7-7b.

Figure 7-7: The regular V-up (a) and a variation with arms overhead (b).

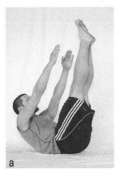
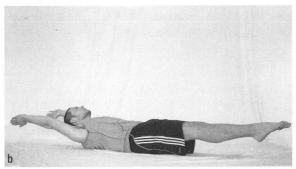

Photos courtesy of Rebekah Ulmer

The windmill

Although many mistake the windmill for a side bend, it isn't. This movement blends hip flexion and thoracic rotation, which means the hips support the load, not the low back. The windmill is a heavy-hitting rotational core exercise, but you must approach it with caution. Don't rush weight onto this movement. First, practice the windmill without weight, and then after you perfect the movement pattern, try the windmill with a kettlebell or dumbbell. Here are the steps:

1. **Press the weight overhead and lock it. Then assume a shoulder-width stance, but point your feet at a 45-degree angle away from the weight (see Figure 7-8a).**

   The stance setup is critically important. You must angle your feet away from the weight; otherwise, you won't be able to properly push your hips back and perform the movement.

2. **Start the windmill by pushing your hips back and shifting most of your weight onto your rear leg (the leg under the weight; see Figure 7-8b).**

   You should displace approximately 75 percent or more of your weight to your hind leg. If this isn't the case, you need to work on pushing your hips back further.

3. **As you start to bend at the hips, look up at the bell, slightly rotate your torso, and use your free arm to guide you into the windmill by tracking it down your front leg (on the inside of your thigh; see Figure 7-8c).**

   Only go as low as you're comfortable with the windmill, and be sure to keep your eye on the weight at all times.

4. **To come out of the windmill, squeeze your butt, drive your hips forward, and follow the same path in reverse.**

The windmill offers the added benefit of stretching the low back. Light windmills are a great way to loosen up a tight back.

Figure 7-8:
When doing the windmill, make sure the hips support the load, not the back.

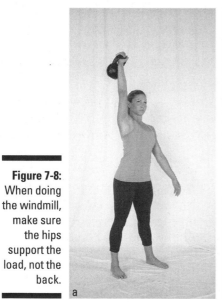
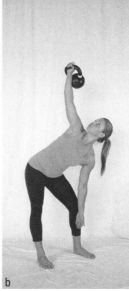
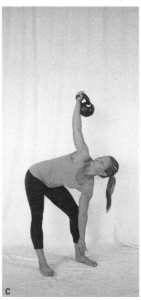

a   b   c

Photos courtesy of Rebekah Ulmer

Intermediate Ab Exercises

In this section, we introduce our first hanging movement, the hanging knee raise, which is the next step in the progression toward what we believe to be the most effective and brutalizing ab exercise in existence, the hanging leg raise (see the later section for this exercise).

We also introduce you to two challenging plank variations that incorporate a rotary stability challenge (the ability to resist rotation). Be sure you master all the beginner exercises before moving on to the intermediate section.

The hanging knee raise

For this movement, you need something to hang off of. A pull-up bar is the obvious first choice, but a set of gymnastic rings or any other sort of hanging device will work well.

The hanging knee raise works the entire abdominal wall — the upper, the middle, and the lower. It's easy on the back and really helps develop the strength needed to complete a full hanging leg raise. The following steps walk you through the hanging knee raise:

1. **Assume a dead hang position (see Chapter 6) from a pull-up bar or rings. Brace your abs and flatten the arch out of your back — think about trying to mimic the "hollow position" from the V-up (see earlier section and check out Figure 7-9a).**

   Try not to use any momentum when performing the hanging knee raise — that means no swinging or kipping! Keep space between your shoulders and your ears while hanging.

2. **Slowly raise your knees up toward your chest, but don't lean back. Instead, try to keep your torso as vertical as possible throughout the entire movement (see Figure 7-9b).**

   This step is often what makes the hanging knee raise and hanging leg raise so difficult but so effective for strengthening the abs.

   At the top of the hanging knee raise, your shoulders should still be positioned close to your ears. If they've gotten too far away, you're probably leaning back too much.

3. **Slowly lower your knees all the way back down and repeat.**

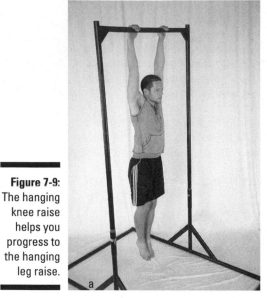 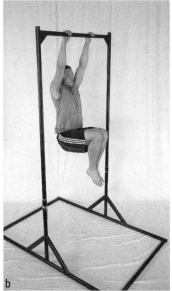

Figure 7-9:
The hanging
knee raise
helps you
progress to
the hanging
leg raise.

a

b

Photos courtesy of Rebekah Ulmer

The two-point plank

The two-point plank brings in an anti-rotational component as well as a balance challenge. For this movement to happen, you must keep everything tight, so expect a full-body challenge as well as an ample burn in the midsection.

Here's how to do the two-point plank:

1. **Assume a four-point plank position (see earlier section), but start with your feet approximately shoulder-width apart.**

2. **Lift one leg a couple inches off the ground. Keep the leg straight.**

   Your alignment shouldn't change when you lift your leg off the ground. If something changes, reset and try again.

3. **When you feel stable with a leg off the ground, slowly raise the opposite arm straight up overhead (see Figure 7-10).**

   The torso and the hips shouldn't rotate when you enter into a two-point plank. Ideally, everything is aligned precisely how it would be if you had all four limbs on the ground.

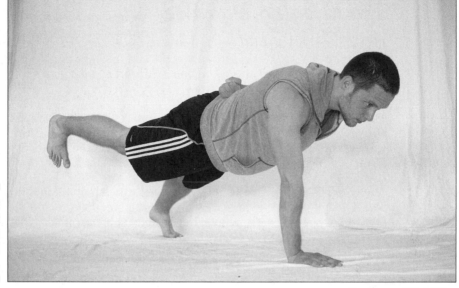

Figure 7-10:
A two-point
plank works
the full
body.

It's best to work into the two-point plank by first mastering a three-point plank off of each limb. For example, hold a four-point plank and slowly raise each limb off the ground, one at a time, for a count of five.

Advanced Ab Exercises

The two movements in this section are both hanging ab exercises. And unless you're a practiced gymnast, you'll likely find both of these movements exceptionally difficult at first. The effort to master these movements is intense, but the rewards that follow are great. Most people who can perform either of these two movements have a strong, hard-hitting, and functional set of abs.

All the exercises that we roll out in the beginner and intermediate sections earlier in this chapter are designed to prepare you for the advanced ab exercises: the hanging leg raise and the windshield wiper. But don't think — even after training extensively with all the preceding exercises — that your first attempt at either of these two movements will be easy.

The hanging leg raise

Almost nobody's first hanging leg raise looks even remotely passable, and that's okay. Over time, as the abdominal wall thickens and strengthens as well as the hip flexors, this movement will start to take on a sort of elegance that few other exercises exhibit.

The hanging leg raise is a staple in gymnastics training, which should give you an idea as to the kind of strength it builds. It blasts the entire abdominal wall — nothing escapes it. Not to mention, it strengthens the hip flexors, the back, and the grip. We truly believe it is the ultimate ab exercise.

The hanging leg raise is the ability to hang from a bar and fold yourself in half. This movement requires not only a great deal of strength but also a lot of flexibility. When most people first attempt this movement, they have a tendency to lean back or to swing their legs up to compensate for their lack of strength, flexibility, or both. Although both of these options make the movement easier, you should try to avoid them.

Here's how to do the hanging leg raise:

1. **Hang from a pull-up bar (or a set of gymnastic rings) with a shoulder-width grip. Tighten everything up as if you're in a plank position and flatten the arch out of your back (see Figure 7-11a).**

   Flattening your back will help prevent using sway or momentum to complete the movement.

   From time to time, you may want to experiment with various grip positions. Occasionally, you can try the hanging leg raise with a narrower grip (hands together) or a wider grip (outside shoulder-width).

2. **Without leaning back or bending your elbows, raise your toes up toward the bar (see Figure 7-11b).**

   Think of trying to "pull the bar to your feet" throughout the movement. Doing so will help engage your lats (armpit muscles) and supercharge your abs.

3. **When your feet reach eye level, lean slightly back if you have to but only as much as you need to (see Figure 7-11c).**

   The hanging leg raise is complete when your feet reach your hands. It should almost look like you're performing a toe-touch stretch.

4. **Lower your legs back down in a slow and controlled manner, and repeat.**

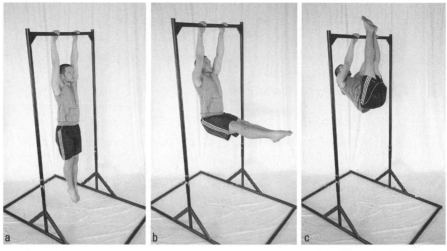

Figure 7-11:
The hanging
leg raise
builds
strength
like you
wouldn't
believe.

Photos courtesy of Rebekah Ulmer

To make this movement easier, first bend your knees before using momentum or leaning back. The more knee bend, the easier the movement, which is why the hanging knee raise is the first step toward the full hanging leg raise. So to progress toward the full hanging leg raise, slowly start to extend your knees further and further until you have achieved full extension. This may take a while, but it works.

The windshield wiper

The windshield wiper is a pseudo hanging leg raise, adding in a fierce rotational component. (*Note:* You must achieve the hanging leg raise in the previous section before you can do the windshield wiper.) The benefits of the windshield wiper are vast, especially for those seeking rotation power and a ripped up midsection. You'll feel this movement across your entire abdominal wall, and we say *across* purposefully because you'll specifically feel its effects around the finger-like muscles of the rib cage (the *serratus anterior*).

Follow these steps for the windshield wiper:

1. **Perform a full hanging leg raise (see previous section), bringing your feet all the way up to the bar.**

2. **Lean back so your torso is horiztonal to the ground and your legs are pointed straight up (see Figure 7-12a).**

Ideally, your legs and your torso should be at a 90-degree angle at the start of the windshield wiper. Do your best to keep your elbows locked throughout this movement.

3. **Slowly lower your legs to one side while keeping your torso facing upward (see Figure 7-12b).**

   Take the movement slow at first! If you throw your legs around too quickly, before you're conditioned for the movement, you may injure your shoulders or back.

4. **Raise your legs back up to the starting position and then lower them to the other side. Bring them back up to the starting position once more to complete the movement.**

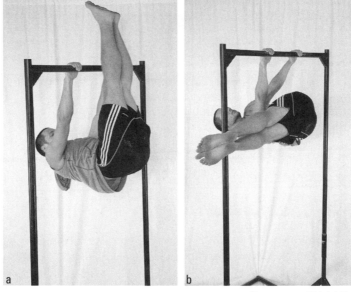

Figure 7-12:
The windshield wiper starts with a full hanging leg raise then rotates.

a

b

Photos courtesy of Rebekah Ulmer

Carrying Skill Drill: The Turkish Get-Up Balancing Act

You're probably thinking, "Why do I need a skill drill for carrying; it's already so simple!" Well, you're right, at least in part. But even with the simplest movements, a multitude of nuances exist — nuances that are often imperceptible to the untrained eye and far too difficult to explain how to do properly.

So instead of attempting to explain, we give you a self-correcting drill to help you figure out the nuances for yourself. With this skill drill, it's all but impossible to make it through without having gained working order over all the nuances.

Dr. Charlie Weingroff, a world renowned physical therapist, strength coach, and functional movement expert says the get-up mimics all the movements of a child between 0 and 14 months and is very revealing of movement compensation or inefficiencies. In other words, the get-up is not only a diagnostic tool but also a corrective tool.

Now the objective of the Turkish get-up balancing act is to perform a full Turkish get-up (from the ground up; see Chapter 3) while balancing something on your fist. Ideally, whatever you're balancing should rest directly on the front two knuckles of your fist.

This drill forces you to maintain proper alignment throughout the entire get-up; otherwise, the object will fall. This movement is a fun and harmless way to master those pesky little nuances. And because the get-up is so closely related to overhead carrying, this drill will greatly improve your performance in that department.

Following is a list of objects you may want to try to balance on your fist:

✔ A book (try this book!)

✔ A shoe (no, you can't stuff your hand in the shoe)

✔ A plate (if you're daring, put some food on it)

✔ A small cup (filled halfway with water), as shown in Figure 7-13

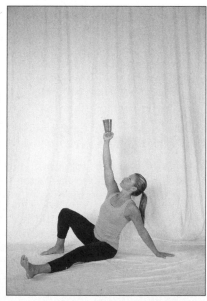

Figure 7-13: When balancing a small cup with water, the worst thing that can happen is that you spill the cup and get a little wet.

Photo courtesy of Rebekah Ulmer

So long as it presents a challenge, any household item will do. What you'll find with this drill is that your overall concentration and bodily awareness will greatly improve.

Core Skill Drill: The Bird Dog

The rudimentary purpose of your core is to protect the spine. The core is a sort of protective mechanism, designed primarily to stabilize and support the spine. Secondarily, its purpose is to mobilize the spine. Unfortunately, most people train only the secondary function — through endless amounts of sit-ups and crunches — and neglect stability work entirely.

Really, a functional core operates at an unconscious level. That is, you shouldn't have to think about stabilizing your spine; it should just be executed automatically. But sometimes even our own hardwiring gets jumbled up, and we suffer a loss of reflexive stability.

In this section, we show you our favorite drill, the bird dog, to help you regain some of that reflexive stability. You can use this drill by itself or in conjunction with the crawling patterns in Chapter 3.

The bird dog is an easy drill to help prime the core and to wake up any sleepy musculature. In fact, you'd benefit from throwing a few sets of the bird dog into your daily warm-up routine. This movement helps reset reflexive core stability; specifically, it trains the core on how to prevent extension of the spine (overarching your low back or flaring your rib cage out), a common problem seen in planks and overhead presses.

A neutral spinal position (no excessive curvature) allows for the most efficient transmission of force through the spine. You're not only keeping your back safe with a neutral spine but also performing better.

Here are the steps to the bird dog skill drill:

1. **Get down on all fours, knees under hips, and hands under shoulders; be sure your back is flat (see Figure 7-14a).**

2. **Slowly start to extend your arm and opposite leg, until your leg is kicked out fully behind you (toes pointed down and knee locked) and your arm is reaching out with your bicep up next to your ear (see Figure 7-14b).**

    Imagine that you're trying to create as much distance as possible between your reaching hand and heel. If at any time you lose your neutral spine position (your low back overarches or your rib cage flares out), stop, reset, and try again.

3. **Slowly return to the starting position, switch sides, and repeat.**

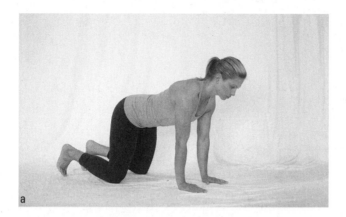

Figure 7-14:
The bird dog
core skill
drill helps
develop
a neutral
spine.

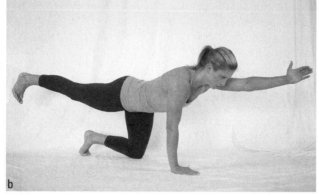

Photos courtesy of Rebekah Ulmer

 Try to stay as relaxed as possible when performing the bird dog. The goal is to get your body to respond automatically (reflexively) to stabilize your position, which you can't achieve if you're tensing too tightly.

Chapter 8

Primal Power Moves for Explosive Athleticism

In This Chapter
▶ Discovering what power training is and how you can benefit from it
▶ Forging dense, durable muscle with the primal power moves
▶ Developing raw, explosive power

*T*he benefits of power training are humungous. Power moves rely on a highly efficient nervous system and perfectly coordinated movement. To express force rapidly is to exhibit movement efficiency, which is a marker of natural athleticism. Power training makes you stronger, leaner, faster, and more robust. It gives you the edge.

That said, precision should always precede power. That's why the movements in this chapter are the last in the series of the primal exercise progressions. They're the true power movements — and by *power,* we mean the ability to rapidly exert force. In previous chapters, we cover explosive movements, such as sprinting, the swing, the clean, and the snatch, but the movements in this chapter require a higher degree of technical proficiency and take the most skill.

All the movements in this chapter are extremely explosive, high-velocity exercises. They build on the skills in Chapters 5, 6, and 7. For example, the swing shows you how to produce and reduce force with your hips, a necessary skill before attempting the broad jump or the box jump, which we introduce in this chapter. The military press and the Turkish get-up (Chapter 3) prepare your shoulders for the overhead demands of the jerk.

If you haven't mastered with confidence all the skills leading up to this chapter, be sure to get comfortable with those skills before proceeding. If you try the movements in this chapter too soon, you may increase the risk of unnecessary injury.

Understanding Primal Power

Primal power is developing power by pushing around heavy things, by jumping, and by sprinting. You don't need any fancy, technical equipment. The good old-fashioned moves work just fine — actually, they work the best.

As we state in the chapter introduction, power is the ability to exert force rapidly. In other words, power is the amount of work you perform in a certain amount of time. So you can increase power in only three ways:

- ✔ Increasing the amount of work you perform over a certain amount of time
- ✔ Performing the same amount of work but decreasing the amount of time it takes you to do it
- ✔ Performing more work in less time

Although power should be your priority when seeking strength, leanness, and athleticism, it shouldn't necessarily come first. You need a solid foundation of mobility, stability, and strength before you start to add in power training. If you train power without the proper foundation, injury isn't a matter of if but when. See Chapters 5, 6, and 7 for exercises to build this foundation.

Your need for speed

The cave man likely engaged in power-based movements on a regular basis. These types of movements were essential to his survival after all. If he wanted to eat, he likely had to sprint to catch his food and even more likely had to spear it (or stone it) then throw it up over his shoulder and haul it back to camp. He couldn't perform these tasks sluggishly.

Humans aren't meant to be slow-moving creatures, at least not all the time. We're designed to sprint, run, jump, throw, and everything in between. For this reason, our muscles are made up of both slow-twitch fibers (for endurance endeavors) and fast-twitch fibers (for short, explosive bouts).

The benefits of power training

Training the fast-twitch fibers, or training in an explosive manner, is quite taxing on the nervous system, especially when you train with weight; therefore, power training offers a very high strength return. Many of the power training movements we explore throughout the rest of the chapter become a blend of heavy strength efforts and elevated cardiovascular stress — meaning you get more work done and burn more calories in less time.

Fast-twitch fibers are also the "look good" muscle fibers, the kind that offer the most grow the quickest and offer the most definition. You can think of them as the mirror muscles because they stand out most vividly when you look into a mirror.

Those who benefit most frequently from power training are athletes. The power moves help them move faster, hit harder, jump higher, and so on. But you don't have to be an athlete to reap these rewards. In other words, you don't have to be an athlete to train like an athlete. Now, we're not saying that everyone should train exactly like an athlete, but everyone can benefit from some elements of training like high-level athletes — power training is one of them.

When training the power movements, you want to minimize fatigue as much as possible. Fatigue slows you down and saps your power. The easiest way to minimize fatigue is to allow as much rest as you need in between sets.

Beginner Power Moves

We start off the power moves with the push press and the broad jump. These movements are both fairly low-skill movements, but they each have their little nuances. Often, the nuances make up movement quality.

With that being said, go easy on yourself with these two movements. They're a starting point, intended to give you the framework needed for the more technical lifts later in this chapter, such as the jerk and the box jump.

The push press

The push press is what people tend to do naturally when attempting to press a weight that's too heavy for them — they use their legs to help drive it up. The difference with this power movement is that you do the leg drive intentionally, not out of desperation.

The push press shows you how to generate force from the ground and transfer it through your body and up overhead. You often see movements similar to the push press, such as the Viking push press, in strongman competitions because it's a clear demonstration of upper body power and work capacity as well as a developer of both.

The *groove,* or path of the weight, with the push press is slightly different from the military press (see Chapter 6). Because you're driving the weight up more so from your lower body than your upper body, the path should be more vertical, or straight up and down, instead of arcing slightly outward. Other than that, if you have a solid military press, you should be able to master the push press in no time. Simply follow these steps:

1. **Clean a weight (either a kettlebell or dumbbell) up into the rack position (see Chapter 5 for cleaning techniques and check out Figure 8-1a).**

   Keep your forearm vertical in the rack position, not angled, to ensure a smooth transition into the overhead lockout.

2. **Dip down, slightly bending your knees (see Figure 8-1b).**

   It's okay if your knees come forward here because you're performing a dip, not a squat; just be sure you don't dip too low — dip just enough but not a smidgeon more. Doing so will diminish your power and fatigue your quads prematurely.

3. **Immediately reverse the dip, driving your heel hard into the ground and imagine that you're trying to jump the weight up overhead. Catch the weight overhead in a full lockout position (see Figure 8-1c).**

   The bell should float up overhead from the drive of your lower body. The arm assists, but the legs do most of the work.

4. **Let the weight drop back down into the rack quickly (don't resist it) and catch it softly by re-entering the dip.**

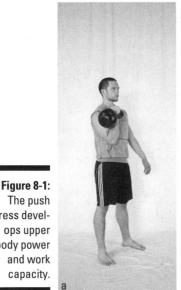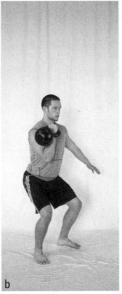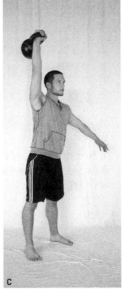

Figure 8-1:
The push press develops upper body power and work capacity.

a   b   c

Photos courtesy of Rebekah Ulmer

The broad jump

If, for any reason, you have issues with jumping — whether it be knee-, back-, or hip-related — don't jump! And if you have prominent movement restrictions or dysfunction, especially with your squatting or hinging, then jumping probably isn't the best option for you. Stick with the lower impact variations until your movement quality improves. If you don't have any issues with jumping and want to keep it that way, then pay very close attention to everything we say in this section.

Jumping is a necessary endeavor in almost all sports and other recreational activities, so it's important to know how to jump properly. Jumping is a tremendous tool for developing explosive lower body power and improving the rate of force production.

The broad jump is an outward jump, or a distance jump (think jumping across a stream); it's not a vertical leap. The movement that most closely mimics the broad jump is the kettlebell swing because you direct the force outward. In fact, you can think of your kettlebell swing almost like a broad jump where you don't leave the ground. See Chapter 5 for details on the kettlebell swing.

Here are the steps to the broad jump:

1. **Assume a shoulder-width stance; initiate the jump by hinging at your hips, just like you would a kettlebell swing, and throwing your arms back behind you (see Figure 8-2a).**

2. **Explode forward (don't forget to swing your arms!) and spring off the balls of your feet; let the sway of your arms guide the movement (see Figure 8-2b).**

   Be sure to synchronize your arm swing with your hip hinge. You'll have to experiment a little with the amount of torso lean in your jump to find that "just right" position.

3. **When you land, make contact first with the balls of your feet (your feet should land slightly apart) and roll gently back onto your heels and into a partial position to disperse the impact (see Figure 8-2c).**

   Whatever you do, *don't* lock your knees because they act as natural shock absorbers.

If anything feels wrong with the broad jump, stop immediately. Pain is your body's way of telling you that you're doing something wrong.

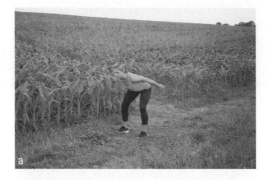

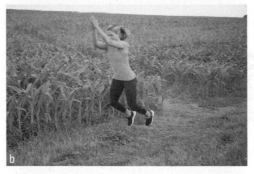

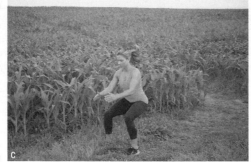

Figure 8-2:
Your feet
leave the
ground and
land on
the ground
together
with the
broad jump.

Photos courtesy of Rebekah Ulmer

Intermediate Power Moves

You can expect to spend a considerable amount of time working out the technical nuances of the two movements in this section: the jerk and the box jump.

These two colossal power and speed exercises are both technical and delicate. Even the most minor infraction, or incongruence, impedes performance.

These two movements develop much more than force production. They show you how to move rapidly and how to do so with eloquence. Think of an Olympic lifter who snatches or jerks a barbell; the movement is so fluid it could almost be described as romantic.

Although we don't show you barbell cleans, jerks, snatches, or any other Olympic lifts in this book, the variations we show you (which you use with kettlebells, dumbbells, or other weights of the sort) offer nearly identical benefits, are quicker to learn, and come with a lower risk for injury.

Olympic lifting is a highly technical skill, and anyone who wants to get into Olympic lifting should start by seeking out a highly qualified Olympic lifting coach. For the rest of you, keep reading.

The jerk

The jerk was originally intended for a single purpose: to heave the most weight overhead as humanly possible. And although that's still a commendable purpose, the jerk has since taken on many other useful functions. When performed with a lighter load and for higher repetitions, the jerk not only remains a great power developer but also challenges the cardiovascular system.

Kettlebell sport (called *Girevoy sport*), which is much more popular in Western culture than in the United States, features high-repetition jerks (often performed for ten minutes at a time) as a competitive event. The power, muscularity, and fluid movement of these competitors are a testament to the effectiveness of high-repetition jerks for building a truly remarkable physique.

With that being said, we highly encourage you to perform your jerks with a kettlebell because it lends itself perfectly for the movement. But if you don't have a kettlebell handy, a dumbbell will work fine as well.

The jerk starts out as a push press (see earlier section in this chapter) but adds in a second dip (or quarter squat) where the lifter attempts to "sneak under the weight." The idea here is that by moving your body under the weight, you shorten the distance the weight has to travel; and the less distance the weight has to travel, the more weight you should be able to lift. Makes sense, right?

Follow these steps to do the jerk:

1. **Clean the weight up into the rack position and assume a shoulder-width stance. Start the jerk the same way you would a push press, by taking a shallow dip (see Figure 8-3a).**

   Don't take long to get into the dip. Think "quick down, quick up," like a spring!

2. **Explode out of the dip exactly how you would a push press. As the weight is accelerating upward, shoot your hips back and land your weight back onto your heels (see Figure 8-3b), coming into a quarter squat position to "sneak under the weight" and catching the weight overhead in a full lockout position (see Figure 8-3c).**

   It's okay if your heels leave the ground during the upward portion of the jerk, but they should be planted when you shoot your hips back to catch the weight.

3. **Stand up out of the quarter squat with the weight locked out overhead to complete the repetition (see Figure 8-3d). Let the weight fall quickly back into the rack position (catch it softly with a dip if you need to) and repeat.**

Figure 8-3:
The easy way to learn the jerk is with patience. Keep practicing and you'll find the groove.

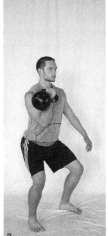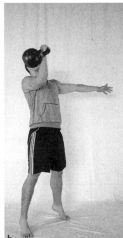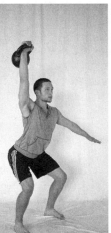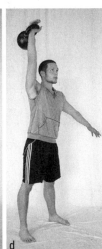

Photos courtesy of Rebekah Ulmer

The box jump

The box jump takes some of the impact out of jumping because you're landing on an elevated surface. So then why do we put the box jump in the intermediate section and the broad jump in the beginner section, you ask? We've done so because you need to develop proper landing mechanics before anything else, and the broad jump is a great way to do that.

Although the box jump is a bit more forgiving than the broad jump, it's equally challenging and offers its own unique benefits. For one, the box jump helps you develop *stand-still explosiveness* — the ability to rapidly "turn it on." Like the broad jump, the box jump helps you increase your natural rate of force production. The box jump is more of a vertical leap, whereas the broad jump is horizontal. Simply put, you jump *up* with the box jump, and you jump *out* with the broad jump. The projection of force with the box jump is more like the snatch, while the broad jump is more like the swing.

When working the box jump, keep the box you're using at or under 36 inches. Higher box jumps ultimately become more of a function of hip mobility than actual explosiveness, and the marginal benefits to be had from leaping to such heights don't merit the additional risks.

The following steps walk you through the box jump:

1. **Set up slightly behind the box or surface you're leaping onto, and assume your natural jumping stance. Initiate the jump by squatting slightly downward, taking a shallow dip (see Figure 8-4a).**

   Here's one way the movement differs from the broad jump. When leaping upward, your take-off comes out of something more like a shallow dip than a hinge.

2. **Explode out of the dip, leaping up onto the box (see Figure 8-4b).**

   The goal is to stick the landing softly, like a cat, with some knee bend and both feet landing simultaneously. Essentially, you should land in almost the exact some position you took off from. If you're landing in a very deep squat, you're probably using too high of a box.

3. **Step — don't jump — down from the box.**

   Jumping down from the box has little benefit and can cause injury.

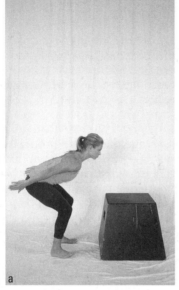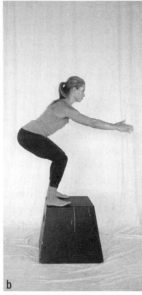

Figure 8-4: Use a box under 36 inches when performing the box jump.

a   b

Photos courtesy of Rebekah Ulmer

Advanced Power Moves

In this section, we show you the double jerk and the double snatch. Both of these movements ultimately land the weight in the same overhead position as the jerk or military press, but each of them takes a distinctly different method of getting it there.

What's great about these double techniques is that they're nearly identical to their single technique counterparts, save a few minor tweaks here and there. All you really need to do is add more power. So if you master techniques in progression of difficulty/power, you should be able to pick up these advanced movements more quickly and easily. That said, don't hesitate to review the single techniques before jumping in to the advanced moves in this section.

For as explosive as the double jerk and double snatch are, they're both relatively low impact. Neither movement — which are best performed with either a set of kettlebells or dumbbells, by the way — has you leaving the ground. So although these movements are advanced, chances are they're still viable options to develop power for those who haven't been cleared for high-impact exercises.

The double jerk

The double jerk basically involves cleaning two weights up into the rack position then blasting them up overhead. Like the jerk, which we show you earlier in this chapter, the double jerk may serve multiple purposes. You can use it for pure power and strength generation (lifting the most possible weight overhead), or you can use it for strength endurance and metabolic purposes (lifting weight overhead for multiple repetitions).

What makes the double jerk so special is that when you combine it with the clean (which you'll do most of the time), it works just about every single pushing and pulling muscle in the entire body. It's as comprehensive as an exercise can possibly get.

When you perform the jerk consecutively (without cleaning the weight between each repetition) it's referred to as *short-cycle*. When you perform a clean between each repetition of the jerk, it's referred to as *long-cycle*.

Here's how to do the double jerk:

1. **Clean two kettlebells or dumbbells up into the rack position (see Figure 8-5a) and initiate the double jerk the same way you would the single jerk by taking a shallow dip (see earlier section and check out Figure 8-5b).**

   Don't waste any more time down in the dip than you have to. The more time you spend in the dip, the more fatigued your legs will become, and the less power you'll have.

2. **Explode out of the dip, launching the bells upward.**

   As you explode out of the dip, think "jump the weight up."

3. **As the weight soars upward, shoot your hips back to "sneak under it," achieving a full lockout overhead and landing in a quarter squat position (see Figure 8-5c).**

   Be explosive when shooting your hips back into the quarter squat and shift the majority of your weight onto your heels.

4. **Stand up out of the quarter squat while keeping the weight locked out overhead to complete the movement, as shown in Figure 8-5d.**

5. **Rise up onto your tippy toes to meet the weight halfway as you let it drop back down into the rack position.**

   You may want to further cushion the impact by landing again in a shallow dip.

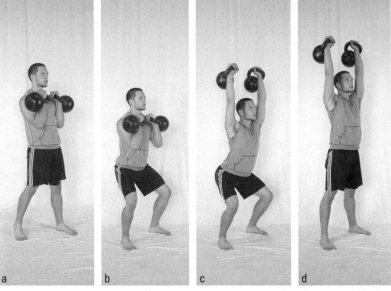

Photos courtesy of Rebekah Ulmer

The double snatch

The double snatch is identical to the single snatch with the exception of stance width (just wide enough to accommodate the weight).

Simply put, the double snatch is a power bomb. You rip the weight off the ground, swing it between your legs, and explode it up overhead in one smooth, uninterrupted fashion. Completing this movement is a commendable effort to say the least.

The double snatch develops hip drive (an athlete's engine) like nothing before it. Except for high-level Olympic lifting, the double snatch is perhaps the ultimate exercise for developing explosive power. It's quite a heinous conditioning tool as well. Think you're ready to give it a go? Follow these steps:

1. **Set up precisely how you would for a kettlebell swing (see Chapter 5), with a stance just wide enough to accommodate both weights (either two kettlebells or two dumbbells).**

2. **Start with a forceful hike back (see Figure 8-6a).**

   This movement isn't a dead snatch, where you rip the weight straight from the ground, so be sure to start each rep with a strong hike back.

3. Explode out of the hinge, standing up as quickly as possible (think "jump," but keep your heels on the ground).

4. Let your elbows bend slightly to guide the path of the weight upward, but don't let the weight arc out too wildly (see Figure 8-6b).

5. As the bells approach eye level, begin to "punch through" into the overhead lockout position. Bring the weights back down into the rack position before throwing them into another backswing and repeating the movement.

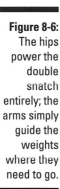

Figure 8-6:
The hips power the double snatch entirely; the arms simply guide the weights where they need to go.

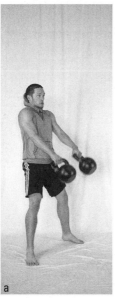
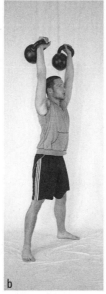

a   b

Photos courtesy of Rebekah Ulmer

Part III

The Paleo Fitness Foundational Program

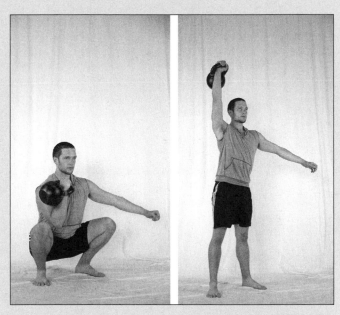

Photos courtesy of Rebekah Ulmer

Visit www.dummies.com/extras/paleoworkouts for an additional intense workout routine that will boost your strength and endurance.

In this part . . .

- Understand the neurological science behind getting strong and build strength, not bulk.

- Discover the truth about cardio, and realize that doing too much cardio can do more harm than good.

- Find out what metabolic conditioning is, why it's so effective at burning fat and building muscle, and how to incorporate it into your own fitness program.

- Create a successful workout program that helps you realize your fitness goals.

- Jump in to Paleo fitness with the 21-Day Primal Quick Start program and then move on to the 90-Day Primal Body Transformation — both complete with detailed workouts and step-by-step exercise instructions.

Chapter 9

The Truth about Strength Training and Cardio

*E*verything has a "truth" nowadays. Ironically, most of the time that truth comes off as entirely untrue. So in this chapter, we give you the truth about the truth.

We can't make any big promises, just the refreshment of the truth in its plainest form. When it comes to fitness, the number of misconceptions about fat loss is surpassed only by the number of misconceptions about strength training. Surely you've heard most of them by now: "Strength training makes you bulky," "Strength training is bad for the joints," and "Strength training stunts your growth." How this bunkum ever gained ground is beyond us, but we assure you, none of it is true.

Conventional cardio is also greatly misunderstood, not to mention highly overrated, and often times abused far beyond the point where it gives any profitable return. In fact, if you moved in the exact opposite direction of "conventional fitness wisdom," chances are you'd be pretty fit! You'll understand what we mean as you work your way through this chapter; all we ask is that you proceed with an open mind.

Introducing Primal Strength Training

Plainly, this chapter is about making you strong(er). In this section, we demystify the domain of strength training and trot out the primal strength-training philosophy, which may be couched conveniently in the following sentence: To get strong, lift heavy.

We define what *heavy* is shortly, but for now, just know that rarely is it anything pink or rubbery. Don't let this intimidate you. Heavy lifting is by no means a dangerous endeavor — assuming you're a healthy individual — unless you go about it unwisely. As with anything else, proper execution is key, which is why we spend so much time in Part II driving proper form into your head like railway spikes.

In the following sections, we outline the different types of strength training, give you the benefits of following the primal strength-training approach, and explain how heavy is heavy enough.

Defining strength training

Strength comes in many forms and extends far beyond the realm of hoisting weight overhead. Although working against resistance is a true test and demonstration of strength, strength is much more than that and serves a much greater purpose than simply allowing you to "lift weights."

Here are a few of the many types of strength:

- ✔ **Limit** or **absolute strength** measures the most force you can exert for a single repetition. A one-rep maximum dead lift is an example of limit strength.

- ✔ **Strength endurance** is your ability to exert a submaximal force over a prolonged period of time. An example of strength endurance is performing push-ups for 30 to 60 seconds.

- ✔ **Power** is your ability to exert force rapidly, such as in the jerk or the snatch (see Chapter 8).

It's important to know the difference between these strength qualities. It's also important to understand that increasing your limit strength will almost invariably increase your strength endurance and power output as well.

The cave man likely didn't have any sort of planned heavy lifting routine, but he probably engaged in some heavy lifting almost every day. And that's what sets apart the primal strength-training approach from most others. Following the primal strength approach, you do a little heavy lifting *almost* every day. That's just enough to get the job done, not a smidgen more.

Strength is cumulative. Strength is more a function of volume (the total amount of work you perform) rather than a function of density (how much work you perform in a fixed period of time, such as a day, an hour, or a set). Therefore, you'll likely get just as strong — if not the teensiest bit stronger — by performing ten reps a day spread out over seven days than by performing 70 reps all in one day.

Acknowledging the benefits of lifting heavy things

No endeavor is more profitable to the body than the effort of lifting heavy things. We can't overstate this. And make no mistake about it: Strength training *is* lifting heavy things. Just because you're lifting weights doesn't necessarily mean you're strength training. In fact, you really don't need any weights to train strength, as you find out through the challenging bodyweight exercises found in Part II.

Aside from the more obvious benefits of looking good with your clothes off and enhanced athletic performance, strength training may also help prevent, reverse, or ward off the symptoms of the following malaises:

- ✔ Arthritis
- ✔ Back problems
- ✔ Depression
- ✔ Diabetes
- ✔ Obesity
- ✔ Osteoporosis

Being strong fixes just about everything. If you struggle with weight issues, getting stronger will help you lean out. If your athletic performance isn't quite where you want it to be, getting stronger will certainly help you with that, too. And if you suffer frequently from injuries, additional strength will amplify your resilience.

Determining how heavy is heavy enough

To get strong, you have to lift heavy, but what exactly is *heavy?* Well, unfortunately, no definite number or weight can define heavy, because *heavy* is a relative term. What may be heavy to you may not be heavy to someone else, such as a gymnast or power lifter.

You have to define your own definition of heavy, and that definition will change as you grow stronger and stronger. The goal, therefore, should always be to make your current heavy light.

To answer the question "what is heavy?" as simply as we can, we say that if you can lift something for more than five repetitions, it's not heavy. So you could say that a "heavy" weight is any weight that you can move one to five times, but no more than that. This definition is what we use to base our strength-training rep range of one to five on. If we go over five reps throughout any of the strength exercises, then we're training something other than limit strength. For example, the push-up may start out as a heavy strength effort, but as you become proficient at it and can perform multiple repetitions, it becomes a strength endurance effort.

The lighter the weight, the more reps you add, and the more you start venturing into strength endurance training.

Differentiating between Strength and Bulk

Certainly, some of the more foolish delusions about strength training are the notions that it will turn you into a sort of Hercules, that it will blow your body out of proportion, so to speak, and that when you stop working out, all that monumental muscle will turn directly into fat. This idea is wrong, dead wrong.

First off, building muscle and building strength are two different operations:

- Building muscle (or bulking up) requires a particular set-and-rep scheme designed primarily to break the muscle down to trigger growth. If you really want to bulk up, you also have to increase calories (a difficult task all its own because you can't make muscle out of nothing, after all).
- Strength training is designed to improve the efficiency of the nervous system — it's not aimed chiefly at breaking down muscle tissue. In fact, muscular fatigue isn't generally desired in strength training as it is in conventional bodybuilding practices.

Even with all of that being said, putting on a lot of muscle is hard work — most men who try can't do it. So if you're afraid of bulking up, rest assured: You'll gain no unwanted bulk here, no matter how strong you get. Instead, you'll develop a lean, dense muscle, like the physique of a gymnast.

To address the last issue in the statement at the beginning of this section, muscle doesn't turn into fat. That's impossible. Muscle is muscle; fat is fat. You can gain muscle, and you can lose muscle. You can gain fat, and you can lose fat. But you can't turn muscle into fat any more than you can turn silver into gold. They are two completely distinct and entirely separate things.

In the following sections, we dig a bit deeper into the differences of strength and bulk by introducing the concept of strength as a habit and explaining that muscle mass is a choice.

Strength is a habit

Strength isn't a result of how muscular you are but rather the consequence of your behavior. A *habit* is something done regularly — so much so that it almost becomes involuntarily. The word *habit* comes from the old French word for "clothing"; so you may think of a habit as something you wear based on your personality.

Strength is merely a habit, you see. And strong people are strong because they've gotten into the *habit* of practicing strength. There's really no mystery to it. If you want to get strong, you must get into the habit of practicing strength — of lifting heavy things from time to time.

Through practice, your body will adapt, tense harder, and grow stronger. It doesn't matter how big or how little you are; you can get strong. All you need to do is practice, practice, practice.

Strength is the ability for your muscles to generate tension, which is controlled by your nervous system, not the size of your muscles. Strength isn't the result of big muscles; it's the result of practice.

Muscle mass is a choice

If you want bigger muscles, we can help you with that, too. But don't let the fear of bulking up stop you from lifting heavy, because that's an entirely illogical and unfounded fear.

If you want to put on some size — either for aesthetic or athletic purposes — we show you how to do so safely in Chapter 16. Just know for now that muscle mass is a choice; you don't have to put on weight to get stronger if you don't want to.

Yes, admittedly some muscle gain is unavoidable when lifting heavy things, but this is something to celebrate, not condemn. When simply doing primal strength training, you'll develop a lean, dense type of muscle, which is very aesthetically pleasing and nothing that can be described as bulky.

Gaining Strength without Gaining Weight

We should have called this section "Gaining Strength *with the Option of* Gaining Weight," because for those of you who want to add some muscle mass, your ability to do so increases in direct proportion to your absolute strength. To say it another way, the stronger you are, the more potential you have to add muscle mass.

The reverse is also true to a large extent; that is, the stronger you are, the more potential you have for total body leanness. Either way, it pays to be strong.

The key to gaining strength isn't found in gaining muscle, although the key to gaining muscle is found in gaining strength. Really, the key to gaining strength is found in gaining movement efficiency, or to put it more succinctly, fine-tuning your nervous system.

Your nervous system is your operations manager; it dictates how hard your muscles are allowed to tense. And tension is strength, loosely speaking. So the harder you can tense a muscle, the more strength you can display.

In the following sections, we explore how to build tension, strength, and relaxation into your normal routine to get the results you want.

Tensing (and relaxing) muscles to develop strength

There are really only two ways to go about generating more tension. The first is to lift more weight. The second is to lift the same weight faster. Both of these options are viable for gaining strength. But there's more to it than that.

The body will allow only so much tension to be generated at any given time. This is a safety mechanism to be sure, designed mostly to protect your joints. But, unfortunately, this mechanism typically kicks in far too soon — long before you're in any real danger of harming yourself from tensing too hard. So you have to teach the nervous system that it's okay to generate more tension, to push back the tension threshold. That is strength.

Flexibility is achieved in much the same way, but instead of teaching the nervous system that it's okay to tense up, you must teach the nervous system that it's okay to relax. And it's between these two spectrums (tension and relaxation) that all human movement lies. It's important to practice both because too much of either one (tension or relaxation) isn't a desirable thing. Ideally, you want to be tense only when you have to be.

While tension is strength, relaxation is speed. Most athletic movements, such as a punch or a jump, are a blend of tension and relaxation.

Combining heavy weight and low reps

The secret to building strength is heavy weight and low reps. If you can work high reps, then the weight you're using isn't heavy enough. Simple as that. You pick a lift — any lift you want — then find a weight you can lift for no more than five repetitions at a time, and then you work multiple sets, resting as much as you need to between each set.

So here's the strength equation you should use to focus your workouts:

>   Strength = Heavy weight + Low reps + Multiple sets

- ✔ *Heavy weight* is relative to you, but you shouldn't be able to lift it for more than five repetitions.
- ✔ A *low rep* range indicates sets of five repetitions or less.
- ✔ *Multiple sets* may be anywhere from 2 to 12 sets, depending on the structure of the program.

This formula is at the heart of each primal fitness program throughout this book. And with a solid understanding of this equation, you can go forth and design your own strength program. But don't worry about that, because we've got you covered there. We just want you to understand the philosophy behind the primal fitness programs, and more importantly, why they work.

Deciding on your training frequency

Training frequency answers the question, "How often should I train?" The answer is, if you want to get stronger, pretty often.

Earlier, we made the assertion that strength is acquired through practice, so wouldn't it make sense then to practice as often as possible? Well, sort of, but not entirely. The human body needs rest. It needs time to recover and to adapt. Rest is done outside of the gym, so more isn't always better in this regard.

Furthermore, you must keep in mind the Paleo fitness principle of doing the absolute least amount to reach your goals. So what's the least amount of practice you need to hit your strength goals? The answer varies per individual, but you'll likely need somewhere between three and five days a week of strength-training practice.

If you're new to weight lifting, gains will come quickly, and you may be able to get away with a little more. If you're a veteran, then you'll likely need more recovery time to get to the next level and would probably do better with less. Either way, the goal should be to practice as much as you have to but as little as you need to.

Working the best strength-building exercises

Are some exercises better suited for building total body strength than others? We think so, yes. Typically, the bigger the movement, the higher the strength return.

For example, the squat is often hailed as the king of all strength-building exercises, with the dead lift trailing closely behind. Both of these movements allow for a tremendous amount of stress (weight) to be put on the system. No other lift allows you to move as much weight as the squat or dead lift.

A classic starter strength-building program may typically be comprised of the following lifts:

- Dead lift
- Squat (either front or back squat)
- Bench press
- Pull-up
- Loaded carry

This list is fairly simple but somewhat lacking. Humans are meant to move in all ways, so don't think you should restrict your strength training to just these five exercises. In fact, you don't even have to worry about selecting the best strength-training exercises because we've already done it for you. All the movements in Part II are our choicest selection of total body strength-building exercises. We carefully chose all the movements we believe offer the biggest bang for your buck (the vital few) and have weeded everything else out. There's nothing superfluous.

But constructing a good exercise program is a lot like building a delicious recipe. The ingredients (exercises) are only part of what makes it successful. The success of a recipe depends largely on the ordering, the pairing, and the preparation of the ingredients. So, too, does the success of an exercise program depend on how you mix, match, and serve the exercises. An exercise program can be overdone and collapse in on itself like an overcooked soufflé, or it can be underdone and fall flat as a biscuit. It's a delicate art.

But you need not concern yourself with any of that, really, because we've prepared the recipes for you and trot them out in Chapters 12 and 13. All you need do is follow them and make sure you master the form.

Leaving the Chronic Cardio Syndrome Behind

Chronic cardio is the nefarious condition of overtraining brought about by an unjustified abundance of steady-state cardiovascular activities. The most common culprit is the treadmill. This condition is communicable, as you can see for yourself should you ever feel the need to walk into a big-box gym again. The treadmills are always *occupado,* swarmed like Porta-potties at a tail gate, but for no really good reason.

Steady-state cardiovascular efforts, such as trudging for hours at a time on a treadmill, offer very poor metabolic return. To put it as delicately as we can, it's just not worth your time, and it's not a coincidence that those who lift weights and engage in short, intense bouts of exercise almost always look and perform better than those who commit themselves solely to the treadmill, elliptical, or bicycle.

It's been proven again and again in scientific circles that short bouts of intense exercise are far more effective for fat loss and overall vitality than long bouts of moderate-intensity exercise have ever been. So throw out the idea that you need to run on a treadmill to lose weight. It's a garbage idea and a wholly ineffective way to go about weight loss and cardiovascular conditioning. The cave man never did this type of exercise and neither should you.

Excessive moderate- to high-intensity cardiovascular activities — often referred to as *steady-state cardio* — creates a *hormonal nightmare* — the result of chronically elevated cortisol levels (or natural stress hormone) that may lead to a plethora of ailments linked to overtraining, such as poor sleep quality, mood swings, loss of libido, joint problems, and injury.

In the following sections, we dig a little deeper into the side effects of excessive cardio, and we explore ways you can use cardio to your benefit, alongside strength training.

Facing the little-known drawbacks of excessive cardio

Excessive steady-state cardio — or excessive moderate-intensity exercise, such as running on a treadmill — is at best a malinvestment of time that could be better spent lifting heavy things or engaging in shorter, more intense forms of exercise (such as metabolic conditioning). At worst (and more likely), it's an investment in your destruction!

Here are some of the drawbacks of excessive cardio:

- Chronic levels of inflammation
- Decreased ability to recover
- Increased free radical production (oxidative damage)
- Increased likelihood of injury
- Joint problems
- Persistently elevated levels of cortisol (stress hormone)

When we say *excessive,* we mean precisely that, but chances are the definition of excessive is probably less than you think. An hour or two of steady-state cardio a day is often more than enough to trigger the deleterious conditions of chronic cardio. Sometimes, it takes even less than that.

Really, all of this should come with a great sigh of relief, because who really enjoys long, trudging runs on the treadmill anyway? We know of very few.

Don't get us wrong: A light, springy jog every now and then is all very well and good. We just prefer you do it outdoors and in minimalist footwear. Moderate-intensity exercise is best performed in as relaxed a state as possible. But rarely do you see people on the treadmill in this state. What takes form on the treadmill can hardly be described as proper running form at all; it's more of a continuously falling motion. The mechanics are heavily distorted, and force isn't properly transmitted. This form wreaks havoc on the joints, so it's no wonder joint pain and other ailments, such as shin splints, are so prevalent amongst those who run on a treadmill.

Doing what you love

Our recommendation for light- to moderate-intensity cardiovascular efforts is simply to do what you love, so long as the activity is relatively light and joyful. If you truly love to run, then run. Just monitor for the signs of chronic cardio, and scale back as needed. Again, we recommend you take your running outdoors and spend plenty of time on mastering proper running mechanics.

If you like basketball, play basketball; if tennis is more of your thing, then tennis it is! Maybe you enjoy Frisbee, which is great because Frisbee is a perfect low-intensity cardiovascular activity. And if you like to cycle, then go cycle (again, just don't overdo it).

The possibilities here are endless, and we even encourage you to experiment, change it up, and try new things. The mind and body thrive on variety (to an extent). And when you begin something new, the excitement of developing new skills often helps motivate you and gets you moving when you otherwise wouldn't. So if you've never tried dancing before, well, now's your chance!

Hiking is a marvelous endeavor, as well as a potent fat burner. Fasted hiking — such as hiking first thing in the morning — is a sneaky little way to shed stubborn body fat. (See the next section for more on fasting.) Hiking is also a relaxing endeavor, offering a sense of tranquility. We can't recommend it enough.

Getting more out of your cardio with fasting

Your body is naturally in a fat-burning state when you wake up, so why not take advantage of this and perform your low-intensity exercise first thing in the morning, right before breakfast!

Even just a brisk, 20-minute walk in a fasted state can yield some seriously impressive fat-loss results, especially when combined with all the other strategies outlined in this book. And don't worry about losing your precious muscle; low-intensity cardiovascular training first thing in the morning, while fasted, selectively destroys body fat, leaving your lean muscle practically untouched. Just be sure to keep the intensity low enough — that is, at a level of exertion where you can comfortably hold a conversation.

When performed in a fasted state, all the positive effects of exercise are amplified (both low-intensity and high-intensity). This combination is potent for not only fat loss but also brain function, cellular cleansing, and immune support. Fasting and exercise are perhaps nature's ultimate tonic for longevity.

Chapter 10

Metabolic Conditioning: Burn Fat Like Raw Meat on a Hot Grill

....

....

Short and intense exercise has been proven again and again to be far more effective for burning fat and building muscle than prolonged bouts of moderate-intensity exercise have ever been. So why is it then that people cling so stubbornly to the treadmill, like a tick on a dog, when science tells them there's a better, quicker way of getting the job done?

The answer, in part, lies in the tacky and overblown marketing efforts of the companies responsible for these grandiose pieces of equipment. Surely, you've witnessed the late-night infomercials. The claims are always appealing, always encouraging, and always wrong. And that's because they're based on what's entirely untrue, which is often far more interesting than what *is* true.

The truth is, nothing is inherently appealing or even all that marketable about what really works for fat loss. Hard work is a hard sell; it's much easier to market the "easy button." But you won't find that here, and we offer no apologies.

Paleo fitness is about doing the least amount of work you need to do to get the job done, but we don't promise you that any of that work will be easy. To be frank, what we talk about in this chapter may very well be the most intense form of exercise you've ever experienced.

Heinous, diabolical, merciless, inhumane, and monstrous are just a few of the adjectives used to describe *metabolic conditioning* — the practice of taxing multiple muscle groups and energy systems simultaneously. Get ready to add your own adjectives as you dive into metabolic conditioning in this chapter.

Introducing Metabolic Conditioning

The human body relies on a substance known as ATP (adenosine triphosphate) to supply energy, commonly referred to as the body's "energy currency." The human body can use carbohydrates, fats, and protein to supply itself with this energy currency. *Metabolic conditioning* is any form of exercise aimed to increase your body's efficiency for storing and delivering energy (ATP).

To further understand this process, you must also know that three energy systems, or *metabolic pathways*, in the human body supply ATP:

- ✔ **Phosphagen:** The phosphagen energy system fuels the high-intensity and shortest-lived bouts of movement (typically ten seconds or less), such as the swinging of a baseball bat, a jump over a creek, or the first couple of seconds of a sprint. This system is *anaerobic,* meaning it doesn't require oxygen to fuel metabolism.

- ✔ **Glycolytic:** The glycolytic pathway is the traditional carb pathway that fuels moderately intense and relatively short-lived exercise (lasting only a few minutes). It takes over after the phosphagen system. Also, the conversion of carbs into ATP results in the production of lactate, which leads to that burning sensation in your muscles. This system is also anaerobic.

- ✔ **Oxidative:** The oxidative energy system is the primary endurance system that supports long-term, low-intensity forms of exercise, such as jogging, hiking, and so on. This system is *aerobic,* meaning it uses oxygen to fuel metabolism.

In short, when you increase the efficiency of the various metabolic pathways, you increase your overall work capacity, which in turn leads to the ability to perform a broad range of physical tasks with general competency.

The body responds to stress by becoming more efficient. Strength is a form of efficiency and so is conditioning.

You can use a number of fitness methods for metabolic conditioning. As long as the multiple pathways are all appropriately taxed, you'll achieve the desired effect. A few of the more common approaches include interval training, cross-training, and circuit training. Although these approaches are all very well and good, we prefer an entirely different method altogether. We explore this method in the section "Turbocharging Fat Loss with Complexes," later in this chapter.

Metabolic conditioning, commonly referred to as *metcon,* has been around formally since the 1970s. The name was originally coined by Arthur Jones (the inventor of the Nautilus), who wrote about the amazing benefits of shortening the rest between exercises performed in a circuit (back to back). The following sections go into detail about those benefits and explain why metabolic conditioning is far more effective than traditional cardio for burning fat and building muscle.

Discovering the benefits of metabolic conditioning

Work capacity is your ability to produce and maintain work of various intensities and durations. It's a desirable trait for any type of athlete because when you match sport-specific skills, the sheer ability to outwork your opponent often leads to victory.

And because the direct result of metabolic conditioning is an increase in work capacity, it can literally help you defeat your opponents. Through metabolic conditioning, you'll be able to go harder, go farther, and go longer. Now *that* is a competitive advantage. Moreover, short and intense metcon sessions have a profoundly positive hormonal impact, surging the production of natural growth hormone (that's a good thing).

Too much intense exercise is *not* a good thing, though. In fact, almost all the positive hormonal benefits of intense exercise may be reversed if you push it for too long or too often. In this case, less truly is more.

The miraculous fat-loss effects brought about by metabolic conditioning are likely to interest you the most. Nothing cuts through fat quicker than short, intense metabolic conditioning sessions. And here's why: Short, intense metcon workouts create a huge oxygen debt, also known as *exercise post oxygen consumption* (EPOC) or, informally, the *after-burn effect.* EPOC brings about an elevated and prolonged consumption of fuel — that fuel being calories. It also results in the breakdown of fatty acids into the bloodstream, where, if your body takes proper advantage of it (see the section "Getting results in just 15 minutes"), the fatty acids may then be oxidized (burned off).

So metabolic conditioning results not only in a long-term calorie burn — that is, your metabolism may stay elevated for up to 48 hours post workout, not something you can get through traditional cardiovascular efforts! — but also in the immediate breakdown of stored body fat. In this vulnerable state, fat burning may be swiftly executed by following up your short and intense metcon sessions with low-intensity cardiovascular efforts.

Switching on your fat-burning furnace

If there's an ultimate exercise formula for fat loss, here it is:

> High-intensity metabolic conditioning (short duration) + Low-intensity cardiovascular efforts (moderate to long duration)

The simplest example of this combination is to pair 15 minutes of sprints (a high-intensity form of metabolic work) with 30 to 60 minutes of walking (a low-intensity cardiovascular activity). The goal is to use the power of high-intensity metcon work to drive the fatty acids into the bloodstream and then switch over to the low-intensity cardiovascular efforts to oxidize (burn off) those fatty acids.

Metabolic conditioning alone is primarily an anaerobic endeavor (without oxygen) and doesn't rely heavily on fatty acids for fuel as much as low-intensity aerobics do. The down side to just working aerobics, however, is that you miss out on all the positive hormonal benefits of high-intensity work as well as the huge caloric after-burn. When you combine these efforts — the high and the low — you're truly able to switch on your natural fat-burning furnace.

Instead of eating after a high-intensity workout, go for a brisk 20-minute walk, and then eat. This little tweak can really make a difference in your fat-loss results.

Getting results in just 15 minutes

When you're cooking something, say, a piece of chicken, you typically cook it only until it's done, right? You don't continue to cook it after it's done, because then it's overdone, and that's bad.

You need to approach exercise the very same way. You want to apply just the right amount you need to get the job done and no more. You can easily overdo exercise with metabolic conditioning. And in this case, less is better.

In other words, metabolic conditioning imparts a considerable amount of stress on the system; therefore, you must apply it judiciously. So how much do you need exactly? Well, the answer, as any good coach will tell you, is it depends. And mostly it depends on what you want to achieve.

We provide specific prescriptions for metabolic conditioning based on various goals in Chapters 12 through 14; for now, note that you can typically achieve the best results with as little as 15 minutes of metabolic conditioning! Yes, believe it or not, this stuff is so potent that 15 minutes is usually the most you'll ever need at any one time. We can't imagine anyone will complain about this, though, because you get to spend less time in the gym and more time on other activities you enjoy.

 A good exercise program shouldn't be designed to destroy you and leave you feeling crushed, dismantled, or obliterated. A good exercise program should challenge you but leave you feeling charged, confident, and successful. So even if you feel like you can do a lot more, rarely does that mean you should.

Turbocharging Fat Loss with Complexes

Complexes are a series of exercises you perform successively — flowing from exercise to exercise with little to no rest in between. Complexes are different from circuit training because you typically perform them with a single modality, such as a barbell, dumbbells, a sandbag, your own body weight, or — our personal favorite — a set of kettlebells.

Complex design is a delicate art. It must be constructed in such a way that it allows you to cycle through various muscle groups and energy systems. This way, the system as a whole may be kept under a prolonged period of stress, and no one muscle group is fatigued to the point of failure.

Like most other forms of metabolic conditioning, complexes combine moderate to heavy strength efforts with elevated cardiovascular stress. Complexes keep the kidneys, the heart, and the lungs working hard while stressing various muscle groups and doing so in a super time-efficient manner — very rarely will a complex take more than three minutes to complete.

To keep the body adapting, you'll do some complexes for time and some for reps. You'll do some heavy complexes and some light. You'll do some long complexes and some short. When we get into the primal programs in Chapters 12 and 13, you'll quickly see that there's no shortage of complexes to choose from to keep your metabolic conditioning varied and exciting.

Complexes are best performed with either your own body weight or with kettlebells because they both allow for "flow." Dumbbells are clunky and sometimes hard to handle with the ballistic movements, such as swings, cleans, and snatches, and barbells are far too large, impossible to swing between the legs, and bring with them the added inconvenience of having to load and unload weight plates. However, you *can* do complex work with barbells or dumbbells. And you can adapt any complex we show you throughout this book to dumbbells or barbells, but our top pick remains kettlebells.

Although barbell complexes are possible and can be quite effective, we don't recommend starting out with them. The barbell is a large instrument and commands respect. Poor form with a barbell isn't as easily forgiven as poor form with your own body weight — and the punishments are far more severe.

In the following sections, we show you how to put together beginner complexes that work for you, using just your body weight or stepping it up with a kettlebell.

Starting with basic bodyweight complexes

Think for a moment what a bodyweight complex may look like. As we said earlier, a complex combines strength and cardiovascular efforts, taxing multiple muscle groups and various energy systems. And a complex combines two or more exercises into a series.

We want you to start by taking a minimalistic approach: What two exercises can you combine to form a bodyweight complex? The answer is limitless. Some combinations may be more worthwhile than others, for sure, but the possibilities are limited only by your own imagination.

A simple pairing of push-ups and pull-ups — which you'll see more than occasionally in the primal exercise programs in Chapters 12 and 13 — is a fantastic "starter" complex. Although not the most strenuous complex ever devised, a pairing of five to ten push-ups with five to ten pull-ups will impose a metabolic demand, even more so when you work in the higher repetition range.

Now, what if you added a set of bodyweight squats in there, making the complex five push-ups, five squats, and five pull-ups performed in a row? In this complex, you switch from upper body to lower body and then back to upper body — the prolonged stress of this complex will quickly elevate your heart rate.

Could you add in another five squats after the pull-ups to round out the work ratio between upper body and lower body? Certainly! Or better yet, you could add lunges instead or any other lower body exercise. The complex then becomes five push-ups, five squats, five pull-ups, and ten lunges (five for each leg). Go ahead and give this complex a try. A taxing effort, is it not?

As you can see, complexes are perhaps the ultimate conditioning tool because they allow you to perform an incredible amount of work in a very short time. What we've shown you here is a basic bodyweight complex. We show you a number of other ways you can construct an effective complex in Chapters 11 through 14.

The following lists provide a couple example bodyweight complexes, using six simple exercises: push-ups, pull-ups (perform rows if you're not able to do a pull-up), planks, squats, lunges, and V-ups. These workouts are a shallow sampling of bodyweight complexes but should give you an even greater idea of the true power of complexes.

When training a complex, never go to failure. If at any time your form starts to deteriorate, take a break and start up again when you can resume with good form.

Here's the first example of a beginner bodyweight complex. (***Note:*** When a time is given for an exercise, perform as many reps as possible with good form within that time.)

- ✔ Exercise 1: Plank for 15 seconds (see Chapter 7)
- ✔ Exercise 2: Squats for 15 seconds (see Chapter 5)
- ✔ Exercise 3: Plank for 15 seconds
- ✔ Exercise 4: Push-ups for 15 seconds (see Chapter 6)
- ✔ Exercise 5: Plank for 15 seconds
- ✔ Exercise 6: Mountain climber for 15 seconds

    Note: A mountain climber is a plank where you drive your knees one at a time up to your chest as quickly as you can. See Figure 10-1.

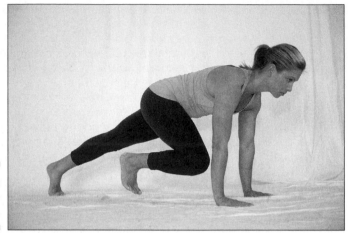

Photo courtesy of Rebekah Ulmer

Figure 10-1:
The mountain climber.

The following beginner bodyweight complex combines exercises for time and some for reps:

- ✔ Exercise 1: Five push-ups
- ✔ Exercise 2: Plank for 15 seconds
- ✔ Exercise 3: Five pull-ups (see Chapter 6)
- ✔ Exercise 4: V-ups for 15 seconds (see Chapter 7)
- ✔ Exercise 5: Five bodyweight squats (see Chapter 5)
- ✔ Exercise 6: Plank for 15 seconds
- ✔ Exercise 7: Ten lunges (five reps each leg; see Chapter 5)
- ✔ Exercise 8: V-ups for 15 seconds

Taking it up a notch with kettlebell complexes

The best device we've ever found for complex work, from the power moves to the heavy strength efforts, is the kettlebell, hands down. The kettlebell allows for "flow" — that is, seamless execution, the ability to hop from exercise to exercise without any hiccups, stumbling, or delay. The compact design of the kettlebell also allows you to swing it between the legs with great ease.

Even though you can select a number of tools to get the same job done, you should always strive to choose the best tool for the job. When it comes to complexes, the kettlebell is king. However, you can adapt any complex to dumbbells or barbells if that's all you got.

Kettlebell complexes typically combine a variety of power movements, such as swings, cleans, snatches, and jerks, and grinding strength movements, such as squats, presses, lunges, and loaded carries. Because the key to metabolic conditioning is found in inefficiency — meaning, variety is your friend — you want to keep the body guessing, or keep it responding to different forms of stress.

The following lists provide a few workouts to play around with, just so you have an idea of what we're talking about. For these complexes, we recommend men use one 16- to 24-kilogram kettlebell and women use one 8- to 12-kilogram kettlebell.

Here's a look at a beginner kettlebell complex:

- ✔ Exercise 1: Two two-arm swings (see Chapter 5)
- ✔ Exercise 2: One goblet squat (see Chapter 5)
- ✔ Exercise 3: Four two-arm swings
- ✔ Exercise 4: Two goblet squats
- ✔ Exercise 5: Six two-arm swings
- ✔ Exercise 6: Three goblet squats
- ✔ Exercise 7: Eight two-arm swings
- ✔ Exercise 8: Four goblet squats
- ✔ Exercise 9: Ten two-arm swings
- ✔ Exercise 10: Five goblet squats

For the next beginner kettlebell complex, perform the complex entirely on your right side first and then switch and repeat immediately on your left:

- ✔ Exercise 1: Five one-arm swings (see Chapter 5)
- ✔ Exercise 2: Five one-arm cleans (see Chapter 5)
- ✔ Exercise 3: Five one-arm military presses (see Chapter 6)
- ✔ Exercise 4: Five reverse lunges (see Chapter 5)

The next beginner kettlebell complex adds in the thruster: Do a squat and then use the momentum out of the squat to go into a press (see Figure 10-2). And, no, using the momentum from the squat here isn't cheating, at least not for metabolic purposes.

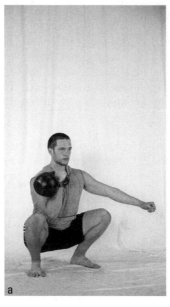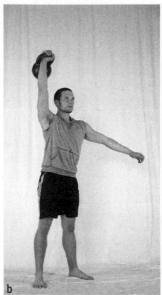

Figure 10-2:
The
thruster.

a

b

Photos courtesy of Rebekah Ulmer

- Exercise 1: Two two-arm swings (see Chapter 5)
- Exercise 2: Two thrusters (see instructions in this section)
- Exercise 3: Four two-arm swings
- Exercise 4: Four thrusters
- Exercise 5: Six two-arm swings
- Exercise 6: Six thrusters
- Exercise 7: Eight two-arm swings
- Exercise 8: Eight thrusters
- Exercise 9: Ten two-arm swings
- Exercise 10: Ten thrusters
- Exercise 11: Eight two-arm swings

- ✔ Exercise 12: Eight thrusters
- ✔ Exercise 13: Six two-arm swings
- ✔ Exercise 14: Six thrusters
- ✔ Exercise 15: Four two-arm swings
- ✔ Exercise 16: Four thrusters
- ✔ Exercise 17: Two two-arm swings
- ✔ Exercise 18: Two thrusters

Here's another complex where you simply alternate between two movements. (***Note:*** To complete this complex, you do a reverse lunge directly into a strict military press, making sure not to use momentum from the lunge.)

- ✔ Exercise 1: Ten alternating lunges (five reps each leg; see Chapter 5)
- ✔ Exercise 2: Ten military presses (see Chapter 6)

To perform the following beginner kettlebell complex, cycle through the three exercises for five rounds without putting the kettlebell down:

- ✔ Exercise 1: One one-arm clean (see Chapter 5)
- ✔ Exercise 2: One squat (see Chapter 5)
- ✔ Exercise 3: One press (see Chapter 6)

So now you have a general idea of what to expect on your metabolic conditioning days. And as you can see, they can be pretty brutal, which again is why less is more!

And don't forget that this is still just the beginning of the beginning; in Chapters 12 and 13, you'll progress toward double kettlebell complexes, utilizing some of the more advanced kettlebell movements, such as the double snatch, the double jerk, and the double front squat.

Chapter 11

Putting Together a Successful Program

Most exercise programs fail because they try to accomplish everything, and by doing so, accomplish nothing. People have the most success when they focus intently on the pursuit of a major goal and put all other minor goals in maintenance mode.

For example, if muscle gain is your goal, pursue muscle gain. Don't attempt to pursue both muscle gain and fat loss at the same time because they are, to a degree, mutually exclusive goals (one requires calorie surplus; the other, a deficit), and will get you nowhere when you chase them simultaneously. Instead, put fat loss on maintenance — that is, keep your body fat levels where they are — while putting on muscle. After you reach your muscle-building goals and are willing to put that into maintenance mode, then you're in a better condition to pursue fat loss.

Make strength a priority. No matter what your goals are — whether they be fat loss, muscle gain, or athletic enhancement — strength assists in all endeavors.

In this chapter, we explain why many fitness programs fail to get you the results you want and introduce some key concepts that are necessary in any successful exercise program. We also look at common questions or concerns when it comes to exercise — whether you're training for strength or fat loss — such as whether you're doing too little or too much and fears about "bulking up."

Understanding Why Most Fitness Programs Fail

Aside from trying to do too much at once — and suffering from a sort of incoherent and illogical busyness — most fitness programs fail because they don't do what's known to work, what has always worked, what's *proven* to work; instead, they elect to practice what's new, exciting, and wrong.

Everything you need to know on how to forge a leaner, stronger, and more athletic physique is already known. Success is not about finding a new way of doing things. It's about finding the *best* way of doing things.

A number of popular fitness atrocities exist today. We don't need to point them out individually, but we outline what makes these approaches unsuccessful in the following sections.

Poor exercise selection

In Part II, we cover the choicest exercises for supreme strength and total body leanness. What makes most popular fitness practices unsuccessful is the complete absence of all these movements and an overemphasis on moderate-intensity cardiovascular efforts (chronic cardio).

Popular fitness programs suffer from a poor exercise selection, so to speak, focusing on the trivial activities that produce only slight results and ignoring the vital few that produce great results. And in the off chance you find any of these lifts in a fitness class in a big-box gym, they're all too often instructed poorly and worked with an insignificant load. There's too much emphasis on reps and muscular endurance and too little emphasis on strength — what really matters.

Unfortunately, too many people unjustly associate sweat with effectiveness. But just because you're sweating doesn't mean that what you're doing is effective. The only way to know whether what you're doing is effective is to pay closer attention to what happens outside of the gym (results) rather than what happens inside of the gym (sweat, burn, and so on).

Lack of a good nutrition program

A number of popular phrases, such as "Abs are made in the kitchen, not in the gym" and "You can't outrun your calories," hint at the notion that no matter how hard you try, you can't out-train a bad diet.

These statements are one version of the truth. But the other version of the truth, the sadder version, is that some people actually can out-train poor nutritional habits, but chances are that person isn't you. And you shouldn't base what you do off the success of the very few. As with most things, exceptions do exist. Some people can get away with things that they shouldn't be able to get away with.

In short, you can expect four times the fat loss results from your training with good nutrition. With poor nutrition, you can expect 1/16 of the results, at best.

If you want to understand the frustration of following a fitness program without first getting your nutrition in order, visit the nearest zoo and watch a monkey chasing after its own fleas. Few attempts are as futile as fitness with bad nutrition.

Here are a few foods you should consider eliminating immediately (for more about proper nutrition and the Paleo diet, see Chapter 15):

- Bread
- Dairy
- Grains
- Industrial seed oils
- Legumes
- Pasta
- Processed and packaged foods
- Soy products
- Sugar (except sugar found naturally in fruits and vegetables)

Some of these selections may come off as shocking, because a number of them are hailed as "healthy choices" by conventional wisdom. But as we've come to know, *conventional* and *wisdom* are two words that when combined often don't make any sense. We go more in depth with this in Part IV and explain why these "healthy choices" may not actually be so healthy.

Inconsistency

The last reason fitness programs fail — even good fitness programs — and surely the most prominent reason is inconsistency. Strict adherence to even a poor exercise program will likely yield better results than loose obedience to a good fitness program. Success is largely a function of consistency.

Inconsistency isn't only an error on the user's end. Some fitness programs are simply set to fail from the start. They're unreasonable — they're far too intense, focused too heavily on the short term, and unsustainable.

We aim to combat this error by providing fitness programs that are flexible and sustainable and that you can fit even into the busiest lifestyle. We also aim to provide fitness programs that are exciting and enjoyable and give you specific strength goals to work toward, to keep you motivated, and to keep you on course.

But ultimately, consistency is a choice — your choice. You're either in or out; we can't do the exercising for you.

Consistency is a habit. It can be developed. And it's developed through the regular practice of those things that will make you successful in your pursuit of health and wellness.

Developing the Recipe for a Good Exercise Program

A good exercise program comes from a well-developed recipe. What we mean is that as long as you understand the ingredients needed for the recipe, you can produce, with a fair amount of consistency, an exercise program that produces predictable and repeatable results.

A fitness program is like a recipe in more than one way. For example, even a cook with very little experience can prepare a decent dish as long as he accurately follows a recipe. And so, too, can a person with very little fitness experience have great results as long as he accurately follows a well-thought-out program.

To construct a successful exercise program, you need ingredients that are simple, sensible, and reasonable. We explain these ingredients in the following sections.

Simple

Simplicity is the key ingredient. The secret to a good exercise program is to strip it down to the fundamentals and leave it at that. The more clutter an exercise program accumulates, the less potent it becomes. Don't let your exercise program look like a teenager's bedroom. Keep it clean.

A good exercise program is neat, tidy, and organized. It's uncluttered. It's not busy solely for the sake of being busy. It focuses on the vital few efforts that produce the biggest results. It ignores the trivial things.

Simplicity also aids in sanity. A cluttered exercise program can feel, and often is, overwhelming, which is no doubt why many people quit. But a simple exercise program is efficient and tidy. It includes only the exercises that allow you to derive the greatest benefit (depending on your goals) and that require the least amount of time necessary for you to reach those goals.

An exercise program improves in direct proportion to the number of things you can keep out of it that needn't be there.

Sensible

Sensible means the program is designed to directly assist you in hitting your goals. It makes sense. It's logical. It has progressions, and, if necessary, regressions.

If your goal is to gain strength, the exercise program should provide a clear, uncluttered path toward that goal. A series of proven progressions should take you from where you are to where you want to be in the quickest time possible.

Many fitness programs aren't designed with an end goal in mind and are too often a hodgepodge of various exercises and modalities, strung together with no apparent rhyme or reason — and so you wind up with a sort of tapioca.

An exercise program shouldn't have in it variety solely for the sake of having variety, any more than it should be busy solely for the sake of being busy. It should, instead, feature the least number of components necessary to get you to your goals. That's efficiency. That's sensibility.

Reasonable

Reasonable means it's something you can handle, especially in the long term. Too many programs burn you out too quickly because they're unsustainable.

The popularity of "insane" fitness programs is surging. Although the idea of working out until you're blue in the face may sound enticing, it's not necessarily such a wise idea, nor is it necessary.

Intense exercise is best served in small to moderate doses. Cellular recovery happens on its own accord and can't be rushed. Not naturally, at least. When you put too much stress on the system for too long — when recovery can't keep up with stress — then you suffer burnout, overtraining, and failure. The problem with unreasonable exercise programs is that although they may work in the short term, they do just as much, if not more, harm than good in the long run due to their unsustainable and insensible practices that put too much strain on both the body and the mind.

You must approach a fitness program thinking of the long term. We recognize doing so isn't such an easy task, because people want results, and they want them quickly. But take a step back before beginning any fitness program, and honestly ask yourself, "Do I see myself doing this program six months from now? A year? Ten years?" If the answer to any of these questions is no, it's time to pause and reconsider what you're doing.

Identifying Whether You're Doing Too Much or Too Little Exercise

When it comes to exercise, it's best to err on the side of caution; that is, always strive to do less, before you do more.

In most cases, people need more recovery time, not more stress (exercise). So if you're not getting the results you want, adding in more exercise may actually be the opposite of what you really need.

An effective exercise program doesn't require you to work out six days a week. Three days a week is all most people need to achieve the results they want, so long as what they're doing is effective and their nutrition is good.

Our recommendation is to stick to something for three months before passing any judgments or making any tweaks. Three months is a fair amount of time to assess the effectiveness of an exercise program.

After three months, and after you've assessed the effectiveness of your current routine, you're in an informed position to either add in or take out an extra day (or two) of exercise. If you make too many tweaks as you go along, you'll never be able to monitor and assess what's actually working. You must control the variables.

Luckily for you, we make this assessment easy with the primal exercise programs in Chapters 12 and 13, giving you specific exercise prescriptions. In the following sections, we help you identify whether you're doing too much or little in your exercise program.

To help assess the effectiveness of your exercise routine, take before photos! Scales can lie, but cameras don't. Before beginning one of the primal exercise programs, snap a few "before photos." Take a few from the front and a few from the side. Then stash those photos for three months. Don't look at them even once! After three months, snap some "after photos," and compare the results to your before photos. We think you'll be more than pleasantly surprised at what you see.

When you're doing too much

Overtraining is a serious matter. It's a prolonged condition brought about when the body is unable to sufficiently recover from the stresses of exercise and often leads to a host of malaises.

Here are a few signs of overtraining:

- Depression/anxiety
- Elevated resting heart rate
- Lack of energy, sluggishness, exhaustion
- Lack of or reverse of progress
- Loss of libido
- Mood swings/irritability
- Weight gain

The simplest piece of advice we can give you is to listen to your body. If you feel overworked and overtired, it's time to rest. "Pushing through it," especially with the aid of stimulants like caffeine, will only make things worse. Rest is the best and the only truly effective therapy in this case.

When you're doing too little

Chances are you know when you're doing too little, because you feel guilty about it — because you know you're skipping out on something you should be doing. Doing too little is rarely the result of an insufficient exercise program — most programs are guilty of prescribing too much. Mainly, doing too little is the direct result of making excuses, which is an error on the user's end.

Yes, a lack of results is a sign that you may be doing too little, but it'd be unfair to make any assumptions without following your exercise program for a good 30 to 90 days. Most people think they can accelerate results by adding in more and more exercise. Up to a point, this may be true, but this strategy typically works only in the short term (if it works at all) and isn't a reasonable, healthy, or sustainable approach to fitness. We don't recommend it.

Motivation, or lack thereof, is usually the problem here. And that's why you should take a little time every day to motivate yourself. That's right — motivate yourself! Don't forget why you started in the first place. Take the time to remind yourself of it every day, multiple times a day.

Also, you may want to find new sources of motivation. As you reach your goals, new motivation is often necessary to get to the next level. Look constantly for new sources of inspiration to give you the push you need.

Overcoming Fitness Roadblocks

Any excuse you make will come true. It will come true because you will make it come true. Making excuses is a habit. The good news is you can break this habit and replace it with other habits that are better suited for a lean, strong, and healthy lifestyle. The excuse-making habit isn't well suited for any sort of productive life.

So replace any excuse-making habits with better habits, such as the habit of consistency, the habit of perseverance, and the habit of personal responsibility. If you want to be successful in your fitness journey, you must be willing to take 100 percent responsibility for yourself.

If you cast blame, you're not taking responsibility for yourself. If you make excuses, you're not taking responsibility for yourself. People who do these things are unsuccessful; so unless you want to be numbered among the unsuccessful, you must act like successful people act, and successful people always take responsibility for themselves.

In the following sections, we respond to many excuses, or roadblocks, people use for not following through with an exercise program.

Too busy to exercise

A few fun sayings handle this objection, most of them hint at something to the effect of "if you don't make time for exercise now, you'll have to make time for the doctor later."

Your health is nothing more than the total of all the decisions you've ever made; that is, every single thing you do can either add to your health or take away from it. Although you can't control everything about your health, you should control everything you can control. To a very large degree, health is a choice. It's a decision. And nobody can decide to be healthy for you.

In this book, we give you the minimalist approach to health and fitness. "No time" or "too busy" is no longer a valid excuse (like it ever has been), especially when some of the workouts featured in the primal exercise programs take as little as 15 minutes.

We've found that when people say they don't have the time, what they really mean is that they don't want to make the time. To that, we say make the time. You'll thank us later.

Feel shaky and tired

Always listen to your body. If something doesn't feel right, stop. Tiredness typically means, believe it or not, that you're tired. Occasionally, you'll get tired, and you just need to back off a little and get some rest.

Chronic tiredness, however, is a more serious problem that we don't have time to talk about in this book, except for the portion of chronic tiredness that may be related to overtraining (see the earlier section "When you're doing too much"). Overdependence on stimulants, particularly caffeine, is a common culprit. Make sure that if you consume coffee, tea, and other caffeinated beverages, you do so judiciously and sparingly.

Also, don't do too much too fast. You have every right to ease into an exercise program, and nobody here is forcing you to do anything. You want to challenge yourself, but you also want to ensure that you're successful. There's no need to push yourself to a breaking point.

Don't want to get too bulky

Although we provide one exercise program to help those who want to put on size, all the other programs in this book give you a sort of wiry strength, a lean, dense, and sculpted look, not a hulky or herculean look.

Keep in mind that putting on size is no easy task, either. Following an exercise program designed to put on muscle mass is only a small part of the equation. Your eating habits are what impart the greatest effect. Putting on "bulk" requires a large surplus of calories. Eating for size isn't an easy task, especially for people who aren't naturally bulky and especially for females.

Lifting heavy doesn't make you bulky. Lifting heavy makes you strong. There's a difference.

Don't have the willpower

People take action for two reasons, and two reasons alone: to seek pleasure, or to get out of pain. No other motives in life exist; therefore, the key to willpower lies in either avoidance to pain or pursuit of pleasure.

People who despise exercise and see it as a pain point unfortunately won't take action and begin an exercise program until the pain of not exercising becomes greater than the pain of exercising. Unfortunately, this pain typically comes in the form of a catastrophe, such as a diabetes diagnosis or a heart attack. We don't recommend that you wait until then to find the willpower to exercise.

If you lack the willpower, you're either not in enough pain — physically or emotionally — to want to seek out exercise, or you don't want the sure rewards that come from exercising bad enough. In other words, you're content with not exercising.

This brings us back to an important point: Take the time to motivate yourself. Go out and actively seek motivation. Find sources of inspiration that make you want to seek out the pleasures to be had from exercising, the sure rewards that come along with a lean, hard, and sexy physique.

Find a picture of a physique you admire, of someone you want to look like. Print it out, frame it, and hang it somewhere you'll see it most frequently throughout the day. Whenever you see it, visualize that physique on yourself. This little trick will help keep you motivated.

Chapter 12

Newbies Start Here:
The 21-Day Primal Quick Start

In This Chapter

▶ Diving into your first primal fitness program

▶ Building baseline strength, conditioning, mobility, and stability

▶ Developing an all-around more resilient, hardened, and leaner physique

*Y*our work begins now.

You *must* be comfortable with all the movements and exercises outlined in Chapters 3 through 8 before moving on to the 21-Day Primal Quick Start program we outline in this chapter. You don't need to be a master at the one-arm push-up, but you should have a solid understanding of proper technique for all the beginner and most of the intermediate exercises. If you don't, take a couple of extra weeks, or as long as you need, to continue practicing these movements.

And, yes, we want you to start with the 21-Day Quick Start, even if you don't think you have to. If you progress too quickly (that is, if you jump to the 90-day program in Chapter 13) before building a strong foundation, you run the risk of acquiring bad habits that may ultimately lead to injury.

In this chapter, we explain what the 21-Day Primal Quick Start program is and what you can expect to get out of it. Then we provide a daily workout and rest schedule for those 21 days. When you're done working through this chapter, you'll be on your way to primal fitness!

Expecting Results Over the Next 21 Days

If you're new to exercise, you can experience enormous and wonderful changes in just 21 days on the Primal Quick Start program. And even if you're a veteran, 21 days is a fair amount of time to realize substantial gains.

If you stick to the program and the nutrition strategies (discussed in Part IV) with an unflagging enthusiasm, you may expect some truly tremendous results over the next 21 days. For starters, you can expect an increase in strength, conditioning, and movement quality and a decrease in body fat. You can also expect the following:

- Greater awareness of your body and a deeper understanding of how all the parts work together as a whole
- A boost in confidence as you monitor your progress (and see results!)
- Workouts that leave you feeling energized, not depleted or beaten
- A challenge that leads to success

Gearing Up for the 21-Day Primal Quick Start Program

On the 21-Day Primal Quick Start program, you work out two days, rest for one day, work out two days, and then rest for two days, and repeat (for three weeks total). Another way to think of it is you work out on Monday, Tuesday, Thursday, and Friday, and rest on the other days. Although the actual days you choose are flexible — you can start Day 1 on Sunday or even Tuesday — we recommend that you mimic the work-to-rest schedule into your week. Broken up into 21 days, this schedule amounts to 12 total days of training and 8 days of rest.

We divide each workout session into strength training and metabolic conditioning, starting with a warm-up — mostly comprised of Turkish get-ups, crawling, and rolling (see Chapter 3 for details on these movements). Metabolic conditioning should always come *after* your strength training — never before it. Most strength-training sessions take no longer than 20 minutes to complete, and most metabolic conditioning sessions take no longer than 15 minutes. So on average, you'll be done with your workout in less than 40 minutes.

Don't forget to add in low-intensity cardiovascular activity throughout your week as much as possible, both on work days and rest days. You can do anything you want for cardio as long as it's lower intensity. Shoot for six to seven hours a week of low-intensity cardio, spread out however you want.

Although you may be taken aback by how simple the strength-training sessions are and may be tempted to do more — don't. We designed the 21-Day Primal Quick Start program to strengthen the following fundamental movement patterns (and subtle variations therein): the push-up (upper body push), pull-up or row (upper body pull), goblet squat (lower body squat), dead lift (lower body hinge), sprinting (locomotion), Turkish get-up (loaded carry), and hanging knee raise (core). We won't stray too far from this structure until after the initial 21 days, and even then, we won't go far from the underlying framework — that is, the overall approach to strength and conditioning.

In the following sections, we explain in more detail what you can expect from the 21-Day Primal Quick Start program and how you should approach each session.

Start with a warm-up

Each work day of the 21-Day Quick Start begins with a warm-up — usually five minutes of unweighted Turkish get-ups and five minutes of crawling and rolling. Here are some tips on doing these warm-ups:

- ✔ To make the most of the Turkish get-up practice, alternate sides with each repetition and go as slow as you possibly can with every repetition. Focus on the integrity of each position of the get-up and don't rush it. See Chapter 3 for more on the Turkish get-up.

- ✔ When crawling and rolling, take your time and have fun. Explore the various crawling and rolling patterns we outline in Chapter 3. Mix it up, and take as long as you need. Five minutes is just a bare minimum starting point.

The combination of Turkish get-ups, crawling, and rolling is the go-to warm-up before any workout. If you feel like you need additional time warming up or stretching, take as long as you need.

Get ready for some repetition

This 21-day quick start gives you baseline strength in a series of fundamental movement patterns. This program is your foundation. It may seem very simple, but that's the point. Variety for the sake of variety isn't a good thing. If you want to develop strength, you have to practice it, which means lots of repetition and little variety.

This simple approach is a low-rep, high-quality set-and-rep scheme and is similar to how a gymnast or a power lifter approaches strength training (arguably the two strongest types of people in the world). When training strength, we rarely suggest doing more than five reps in any given set. Instead, we utilize *ladders,* or escalating sets — where you add reps with each set. A ladder allows you to sensibly accumulate volume (the amount of time you spend under stress or load) without getting too fatigued.

A ladder is comprised of rungs, and each rung has a number of repetitions. For example, most ladders in this book follow either a 1-2-3-1-2-3- or a 1-2-3-4-5-1-2-3-4-5-rep structure. The former is a three-rung ladder; the latter is five-rung. The first rung is one rep, the second rung is two reps, the third rung is three reps, and so on, after which the ladder repeats itself. When working ladders, you rest as long as you need to in between each rung — that is, until you feel fresh and confident that you can perform the next rung with impeccable form.

Be prepared to lift heavy

And now you may be asking, "What weight do I use?" The answer: a heavy one! The weight you use varies from exercise to exercise, but in general, you want to find a weight that challenges you for five repetitions in any given movement. You shouldn't be able to move the weight for more than five repetitions. If five reps is "easy" for you for the bodyweight movements, such as the push-up or pull-up, seek out one of the more challenging variations from Part II, such as the one-arm push up. And if any of the prescribed bodyweight movements are too difficult, regress to an easier variation. For example, if you can't perform pull-ups, do rows.

Don't be so quick to shrug off the basic push-up as "easy" and move on to the more challenging variations. Most people who can bang out 20 reps or more of sloppy push-ups can rarely handle even 5 done properly. Use this 21-Day Primal Quick Start program to dial in your technique and establish quality movement.

The goal is to start the 21-day program with a heavy weight (heavy to you) and to continue to use that exact same weight throughout the entire 21 days. So don't bump up the weight even once over the course of this quick start program, even if it starts to feel light. Only *after* the 21 days should you bump up the weight. We want you to finish these 21 days with the weight you're using starting to feel light.

Expect to improve your conditioning

We keep the metabolic conditioning constantly varied, using complexes, interval training, and sprinting. In this part of the program, you begin pushing the reps into the higher reaches, start feeling the burn, and really start sweating.

As for what weight to use for metabolic conditioning, the general rule is to find a challenging weight for whatever regimen you're doing. Sometimes, you'll need a lighter weight and sometimes a heavier one. Don't be afraid to experiment, and don't feel like you have to go heavy all the time, either — mix it up and wave the load. Occasionally, we may recommend a weight for a particular movement.

Your 21-Day Primal Quick Start

Time to start sweating. Here is your daily workout and rest schedule for the next 21 days.

Day 1

Warm-up

5 minutes of unweighted Turkish get-up practice
5 minutes of crawling and rolling

Strength training

Push-ups: 1-2-3-1-2-3 ladder
Dead lifts: 1-2-3-1-2-3 ladder
Turkish get-ups: 1-2-3-1-2-3 ladder (perform one ladder for each side)

Metabolic conditioning

Four rounds of the following Tabata interval sequence with the two-arm swing:

20 seconds of two-arm swings
10 seconds of rest
20 seconds of two-arm swings
10 seconds of rest
20 seconds of two-arm swings
10 seconds of rest

Note: Tabata intervals are 20 seconds of work followed by 10 seconds of rest. Repeat for four minutes.

Day 2

Warm-up

5 minutes of unweighted Turkish get-up practice
5 minutes of crawling and rolling

Strength training

Pull-ups: 1-2-3-1-2-3 ladder (perform rows if you lack the strength for pull-ups)
Dead lifts: 1-2-3-1-2-3 ladder
Hanging knee raises: 1-2-3-1-2-3 ladder

Metabolic conditioning

Three to five rounds of the following complex:

5 two-arm swings
5 one-arm swings (5 each arm)
5 goblet squats
5 push-ups
30 seconds plank

Day 3 – Off

Day 4

Warm-up

5 minutes of unweighted Turkish get-up practice
5 minutes of crawling and rolling

Strength training

Push-ups: 1-2-3-1-2-3 ladder
Goblet squats: 1-2-3-1-2-3 ladder
V-ups: 1-2-3-1-2-3 ladder

Metabolic conditioning

15 minutes of sprints

Tip: Select a sprinting distance that's challenging but that you can complete — 50 to 75 meters is a fair starting point for most. Run as many rounds with good form as you can in 15 minutes. Be sure to rest as much as you need between rounds so your sprint doesn't turn into a job.

Warning: Sprinting is a super high-velocity movement. Take a few extra minutes to run a few strides and do warm-up rounds before running a full sprint.

Day 5

Warm-up

5 minutes of unweighted Turkish get-up practice
5 minutes of crawling and rolling

Strength training

Pull-ups: 1-2-3-1-2-3 ladder
Dead lifts: 1-2-3-1-2-3 ladder
Hanging knee raises: 1-2-3-1-2-3 ladder

Metabolic conditioning

300 two-arm swings

Tip: Perform these swings as quickly as possible with good form. Divide the sets and reps however you want, and be sure to rest if form starts to sour. We recommend that men use a 16- to 24-kilogram (35- to 52-pound) weight and women use an 8- to 16-kilogram (17- to 35-pound) weight.

Day 6 – Off

Day 7 – Off

Day 8

Warm-up

5 minutes of unweighted Turkish get-up practice
5 minutes of crawling and rolling

Strength training

Turkish get-ups: 1-2-3-1-2-3 ladder
Goblet squats: 1-2-3-4-5-1-2-3-4-5 ladder
Push-ups: 1-2-3-4-5-1-2-3-4-5 ladder

Metabolic conditioning

Three to five rounds of the following complex:

5 one-arm swings (5 each arm)
5 cleans
5 snatches
5 military presses
5 reverse lunges

Tip: Perform the entire complex on your right side first and then immediately on your left. Rest as long as you need to but as little as you have to between rounds.

Day 9

Warm-up

5 minutes of unweighted Turkish get-up practice
5 minutes of crawling and rolling

Strength training

Dead lifts: 1-2-3-4-5-1-2-3-4-5 ladder
Pull-ups: 1-2-3-4-5-1-2-3-4-5 ladder
Hanging knee raises: 1-2-3-4-5-1-2-3-4-5 ladder

Metabolic conditioning

Two rounds of the following exercises:

1 minute of one-arm swings (30 seconds each arm)
1 minute of one-arm cleans (30 seconds each arm)
30 seconds of military presses
1 minute of reverse lunges (alternating legs)
30 seconds of military presses
1 minute of single-leg dead lifts (30 seconds each leg)
30 seconds of two-arm swings
30 seconds of goblet squats
1 minute four-point plank

Tip: Metabolic conditioning isn't just a time to "feel the burn"; it's also a time to work on your technique, or more specifically, to see how your technique holds up under stress. Keep your focus first and foremost on form, and always be sure to maintain poise while under pressure (fatigue).

Day 10 – Off

Day 11

Warm-up

5 minutes of unweighted Turkish get-up practice
5 minutes of crawling and rolling

Strength training

Push-ups: 1-2-3-4-5-1-2-3-4-5 ladder
Goblet squats: 1-2-3-4-5-1-2-3-4-5 ladder
Turkish get-ups: 1-2-3-1-2-3 ladder
120 seconds three-point plank (30 seconds each limb; lift a different limb off the ground each set)

Metabolic conditioning

15 minutes of sprints

Day 12

Warm-up

5 minutes of unweighted Turkish get-up practice
5 minutes of crawling and rolling

Strength training

Pull-ups: 1-2-3-4-5-1-2-3-4-5 ladder
Dead lifts: 1-2-3-4-5-1-2-3-4-5 ladder
Hanging knee raises: 1-2-3-4-5-1-2-3-4-5 ladder

Metabolic conditioning

15 minutes of bear crawl sprints

Tip: Find a long and relatively flat stretch of ground. Pick a distance that provides a good challenge — 25 to 50 meters is a good start — and then work bear crawls (see Chapter 3) as fast as you can for 15 minutes. Rest as long as you need between rounds.

Day 13 – Off

Day 14 – Off

Day 15

Warm-up

5 minutes of unweighted Turkish get-up practice
5 minutes of crawling and rolling

Strength training

Turkish get-ups: 1-2-3-1-2-3 ladder
Goblet squats: 1-2-3-4-5-1-2-3-4-5 ladder
Push-ups: 1-2-3-4-5-1-2-3-4-5 ladder
V-ups: 1-2-3-4-5-1-2-3-4-5 ladder

Metabolic conditioning

Two rounds of the following complex:

2 two-arm swings
2 one-arm swings
2 thrusters (2 reps each side)
4 two-arm swings
4 one-arm swings
4 thrusters
6 two-arm swings
6 one-arm swings
6 thrusters
8 two-arm swings
8 one-arm swings
8 thrusters

Tip: Try to get all the way through the complex without setting the weight down. If form starts to deteriorate, rest immediately.

Day 16

Warm-up

5 minutes of unweighted Turkish get-up practice
5 minutes of crawling and rolling

Strength training

Dead lifts: 1-2-3-1-2-3 ladder
Pull-ups: 1-2-3-1-2-3 ladder
Hanging leg raises: 1-2-3-1-2-3 ladder

Metabolic conditioning

Four rounds of thruster Tabata intervals:

20 seconds of thrusters
10 seconds of rest
20 seconds of thrusters
10 seconds of rest
20 seconds of thrusters

Day 17 – Off

Day 18

Warm-up

5 minutes of unweighted Turkish get-up practice
5 minutes of crawling and rolling

Strength training

Push-ups: 1-2-3-1-2-3 ladder
Goblet squats: 1-2-3-1-2-3 ladder
Turkish get-ups: 1-2-3-1-2-3 ladder
V-ups: 1-2-3-1-2-3 ladder

Metabolic conditioning

20 snatches (10 each side), on the minute, every minute for 15 minutes

Day 19

Warm-up

5 minutes of unweighted Turkish get-up practice
5 minutes of crawling and rolling

Strength training

Pull-ups: 1-2-3-1-2-3 ladder
Dead lifts: 1-2-3-1-2-3 ladder
Hanging knee raises: 1-2-3-1-2-3 ladder

Metabolic conditioning

15 minutes of sprints

Day 20 – Off

Day 21 – Off

Chapter 13

The 90-Day Primal Body Transformation

In This Chapter

▶ Setting goals and tracking progress for 90 days of transformation

▶ Designing your own primal exercise program

▶ Forging a leaner, harder, and stronger physique

*T*he one elementary truth about fitness is that when people fully commit themselves, success is inevitable. So all we're asking here is that you give your all, that you're fully committed, and that you work the full 90-Day Primal Body Transformation program with an unswerving enthusiasm.

Half, or even three-quarter, commitments simply won't suffice. If you're going to do this program, you must be willing to go the whole hog, to completely reinvent yourself from the inside out. Success, like strength, is a habit that you must practice every day.

The 90-Day Primal Body Transformation program is the pinnacle program of this book — and the topic of this chapter — as well as the most demanding and worthwhile. We help you prepare for a successful 90 days by showing you how to build your own 90-day fitness program, with exercises and workouts that challenge you but that you *can* complete. We start off by helping you acknowledge where you are and envision where you want to be after 90 days, and we promise to stand by you throughout the process.

Preparing for Success with Goals and Progress Pictures

Before you begin, we want you to know that we're here for you, both for support and accountability. To prove it, we want you to e-mail us your specific goals and your before and after pictures. Taking before pictures is a proven way to increase motivation and adherence, and taking after pictures, which we refer to more commonly as *progress pictures,* is a great way to keep motivated.

The best way to take before pictures is to wear a bathing suit or tight-fitting fitness apparel, and take one frontal picture (head on) and one profile picture (from the side). Take your before pictures on Day 1, and then take the same poses in your progress pictures every 30 days.

E-mail your goals, your before pictures, your progress pictures, and your success stories to patflynn@chroniclesofstrength.com with the subject line "Primal Body."

Going from Average to Elite in 90 Days

Elite performers are the ones who've moved deeper into the basics. In this program, you'll find repetition, repetition, repetition. The strength training slowly increases in volume (total work performed) over the next 90 days, but the movements themselves won't change, nor will the weight you use.

You will, however, be offered the refreshment of variety with the metabolic conditioning routines. These routines vary from day to day, offering new and exciting challenges. This combination of purposeful, repetitive strength training and variable, high-intensity conditioning will make you a true physical specimen, upgraded in every regard, impervious to damage.

Elements of this program are very tough, so be sure to listen to your body. If you feel too beat to train on any one day, take an extra day off — no big deal. Just be sure it's due to legitimate fatigue and not sheer laziness. There is a stark difference.

Designing Your 90-Day Primal Body Transformation

The ultimate goal of the 90-Day Primal Body Transformation program is to eventually progress through 90 days with the ability to perform all advanced level exercises found in Part II. We highly doubt anyone, save the elite gymnast, is going to be able to do that right off the bat. So start with something that's challenging enough for your first 90 days, and then bump it up each time you do this 90-day program. We explain how to design this program for where you are now and how to progress further in the following sections.

Strength-training exercises

For strength training, you choose a series of exercises — one from each of the fundamental movement chapters in Part II — that are challenging but that also ensure success. In other words, you want to pick exercises that challenge you for five reps but that you *can* do for five reps. (***Note:*** For movements that you don't count by reps, such as planks and carries, consider 15 seconds equal to one rep.) You do these same exercises for 90 days.

After 90 days, you repeat the program with a more challenging set of exercises; however, don't progress onto a more challenging variation at any point *during* the 90 days, even when the variations or weights you've chosen start to feel "easy" or "light." You want to finish this 90-day period with all the "difficult" movements you started out with starting to feel "easy." The next sections walk you through exactly what we mean and provide some example strength-training lineups.

Putting together your strength exercise routine

To build your strength-training routine, select two movements (an "A" movement and a "B" movement) from the chapters in Part II for each movement category (we've listed them here for easy reference):

- **Push:** Push-up, military press, one-arm push-up, bench press, dip, one-arm one-leg push-up, handstand push-up

- **Pull:** Bodyweight row, chin-up, one-arm row, pull-up, L-sit pull-up/chin-up, muscle-up, one-arm chin-up

- **Hinge:** Dead lift, single-leg dead lift, swing, one-arm swing, clean, snatch

- **Squat:** Goblet squat, bodyweight squat, goblet lunge, racked squat, racked lunge, front squat, pistol squat

- **Carry:** Farmer's carry, waiter's carry, racked carry, two-arm waiter's carry, bottoms-up carry, Turkish get-up

- **Core:** Four-point plank, V-up, windmill, hanging knee raise, three-point plank, two-point plank, hanging leg raise, windshield wiper

- **Power:** Push press, broad jump, jerk, box jump, double jerk, double snatch

Throughout this chapter, you'll see references to "double" exercises, like double jerk, double snatch, double front squat, and so on. The "double" simply means you're holding a weight in each hand.

You'll do most of the strength training in a ladder format, beginning with three-rung (1-2-3) ladders and ultimately ending with five-rung (1-2-3-4-5) ladders. Every ladder is comprised of rungs, and each rung is comprised of a number of repetitions. For example, the first rung of a three-rung ladder is one rep, the second rung is two reps, and the third rung is three reps. Be sure to rest as long as you need to between each rung.

The order you do these exercises doesn't really matter, but generally, you should start with the movements or exercises that are most challenging to you. For example, in the daily workouts we outline in the section "Your 90-Day Primal Body Transformation," we list the power movements first, because they tend to require a bit more concentration, but you may perform the exercises in any sequence you desire, as long as you get them all done.

If you're a fitness veteran, you may pick an *advanced* lineup that looks something like this:

- Push A: One-arm push-up
- Push B: Handstand push-up
- Pull A: Muscle-up
- Pull B: One-arm chin-up
- Hinge A: Dead lift
- Hinge B: Single-leg dead lift
- Squat A: Front squat
- Squat B: Pistol squat
- Carry A: Turkish get-up
- Carry B: Bottoms-up carry
- Core A: Hanging leg raise
- Core B: Two-point plank
- Power A: Double snatch
- Power B: Double jerk

If you're somewhere in the middle, you may pick an *intermediate* lineup that looks something like this:

- Push A: Dip
- Push B: Bench press
- Pull A: Pull-up
- Pull B: One-arm row
- Hinge A: Dead lift
- Hinge B: Single-leg dead lift
- Squat A: Front squat
- Squat B: Racked lunge
- Core A: Hanging knee raise
- Core B: Three-point plank
- Power A: Jerk
- Power B: Box jump

And if you're relatively new to fitness or are still working on building strength, a *beginner* lineup may look something like this:

- Push A: Push-up
- Push B: Military press
- Pull A: Bodyweight row
- Pull B: Flexed arm hang (see Chapter 6)
- Hinge A: Dead lift
- Hinge B: Single-leg dead lift
- Squat A: Goblet squat
- Squat B: Goblet lunge
- Core A: Four-point plank
- Core B: V-up
- Power A: Push press
- Power B: Broad jump

Did you notice that we kept the hinges consistent with the dead lift and single-leg dead lift for each level? We recommend you do the same because these two movements allow you to move the most weight. You'll get plenty of the other hinges, such as swings, cleans, and snatches, with your metabolic conditioning.

Now you may very well just take one of these lineups and run with it, or you may design one of your own. The key is to select an exercise or a weight that challenges you for five reps. So if you can perform a bodyweight exercise, such as the push-up, for more than 10 to 15 reps, then it's probably time to move on to a one-arm push-up variation. For the weighted exercises, such as the bench press or front squat, be sure to work with a heavy-enough weight. The dead lift by itself isn't necessarily "advanced," but a 500-pound dead lift probably is.

Choosing a weight that challenges you

The weight you choose for strength training should be something with which you can perform for five reps. If you can move it much more than that, it's likely not heavy enough. Because you do most of the strength-training work in sets of five repetitions or less, it's imperative that you work with a significant load; otherwise, you'll find it difficult to make any significant strength gains.

Like the 21-Day Primal Quick Start program in Chapter 12, you won't increase the weight or move on to a more difficult bodyweight exercise until the 90 days are up. The goal is to start the program with a weight that feels "heavy" and to finish with that same weight feeling "light." Then, after the 90 days are up, you bump the weight up or move on to a more difficult bodyweight exercise, and do 90 days with that weight. This progression takes patience because people are always anxious to progress faster than they ought to. ***Remember:*** You can't rush strength or cellular recovery. It occurs on its own accord. When it comes to strength, patience is a virtue.

Metabolic conditioning

You don't need to worry about building your metabolic conditioning routine; we've got you covered. For each work day of the 90-day program, we prescribe a unique metabolic conditioning routine. All you have to do is select a challenging weight for whatever is prescribed that day (naturally, you'll go lighter on higher-rep complexes and heavier on lower-rep complexes). Other than that, it's all laid out for you.

For the double movements — the double swing, double clean, double (military) press, double front squat, and double snatch — follow the techniques for the single movements but use two kettlebells instead of one. For the double swing, clean, and snatch, adjust your stance so it's wide enough to accommodate the extra bell, but stand only as wide as you need to fit both bells between your legs.

Your daily warm-up

So now that you know what exercises you'll be doing in this 90-day program, you don't want to forget about warming up before each workout. Your daily warm-up consists of five minutes of unweighted Turkish get-ups and five minutes of crawling and rolling (see Chapter 3). The point of the warm-up is to wake the system up, to warm the muscles, and to have fun! Crawl and roll around as much as you need to until you feel limber and energized. Take extra time if you feel the need to stretch, foam roll, or perform any other sort of pre-workout routine.

One of the simplest but most effective warm-ups is to simply perform a few light sets of whatever exercises you're going to be working that day.

Your weekly schedule

This program follows a workout-rest pattern just like the 21-Day Primal Quick Start. You work out for two days, rest for one day, work out for two days, and then rest for two days. Work this pattern into your week however you can, such as the following:

- ✔ Monday: Work out
- ✔ Tuesday: Work out
- ✔ Wednesday: Rest
- ✔ Thursday: Work out
- ✔ Friday: Work out
- ✔ Saturday: Rest
- ✔ Sunday: Rest

Your 90-Day Primal Body Transformation

This is it. You're about to go from zero to awesome in 90 days. You're mentally prepared, and you've made the commitment. Now dive in and have fun!

Day 1

Warm-up

5 minutes of unweighted Turkish get-ups
5 minutes of crawling and rolling

Strength training

Power A: 1-2-3-1-2-3 ladder
Push A: 1-2-3-1-2-3 ladder
Pull A: 1-2-3-1-2-3 ladder
Carry A: 1-2-3 ladder

Remember: Because you don't count carries by reps, consider 15 seconds equal to one rep. So for the three-rung ladder here, you do 15 seconds for the first rung, 30 seconds for the second rung, and 45 seconds for the third rung. The exception to this rule is the Turkish get-up, which you do count in reps.

Metabolic conditioning

Two rounds of the following complex:

2 two-arm swings
1 goblet squat
4 two-arm swings
2 goblet squats
6 two-arm swings
3 goblet squats
8 two-arm swings
4 goblet squats
10 two-arm swings
5 goblet squats

Day 2

Warm-up

5 minutes of unweighted Turkish get-ups
5 minutes of crawling and rolling

Strength training

Power B: 1-2-3-1-2-3 ladder
Push B: 1-2-3-1-2-3 ladder
Pull B: 1-2-3-1-2-3 ladder
Carry B: 1-2-3 ladder

Metabolic conditioning

Four rounds of the following two-arm swing Tabata interval:

20 seconds of two-arm swings
10 seconds of rest
20 seconds of two-arm swings
10 seconds of rest
20 seconds of two-arm swings
10 seconds of rest

Day 3 — Off

Day 4

Warm-up

5 minutes of unweighted Turkish get-ups
5 minutes of crawling and rolling

Strength training

Hinge A: 1-2-3-1-2-3 ladder
Squat A: 1-2-3-1-2-3 ladder
Core A: 1-2-3-1-2-3 ladder

Metabolic conditioning

Three to five rounds of the following complex (perform entirely on your right side first and then immediately repeat on your left):

5 one-arm swings
5 one-arm cleans
5 one-arm snatches
5 one-arm push presses
5 reverse lunges

Day 5

Warm-up

5 minutes of unweighted Turkish get-ups
5 minutes of crawling and rolling

Strength training

Hinge B: 1-2-3-1-2-3 ladder
Squat B: 1-2-3-1-2-3 ladder
Core B: 1-2-3-1-2-3 ladder

Metabolic conditioning

15 minutes of sprints

Day 6 — Off

Day 7 — Off

Day 8

Warm-up

5 minutes of unweighted Turkish get-ups
5 minutes of crawling and rolling

Strength training

Power A: 1-2-3-1-2-3 ladder
Push A: 1-2-3-1-2-3 ladder
Pull A: 1-2-3-1-2-3 ladder
Carry A: 1-2-3 ladder

Metabolic conditioning

100 two-arm swings as quickly as possible with good form

Day 9

Warm-up

5 minutes of unweighted Turkish get-ups
5 minutes of crawling and rolling

Strength training

Power B: 1-2-3-1-2-3 ladder
Push B: 1-2-3-1-2-3 ladder
Pull B: 1-2-3-1-2-3 ladder
Carry B: 1-2-3 ladder

Metabolic conditioning

Three to five rounds of the following complex:

5 double swings
5 double cleans
5 double military presses
5 double front squats

Day 10 — Off

Day 11

Warm-up

5 minutes of unweighted Turkish get-ups
5 minutes of crawling and rolling

Strength training

Hinge A: 1-2-3-1-2-3 ladder
Squat A: 1-2-3-1-2-3 ladder
Core A: 1-2-3-1-2-3 ladder

Metabolic conditioning

15 minutes of bear crawl sprints

Tip: After you're comfortable with the forward bear crawl, try sprinting in various directions — backward, to the left, and to the right.

Day 12

Warm-up

5 minutes of unweighted Turkish get-ups
5 minutes of crawling and rolling

Strength training

Hinge B: 1-2-3-1-2-3 ladder
Squat B: 1-2-3-1-2-3 ladder
Core B: 1-2-3-1-2-3 ladder

Metabolic conditioning

Ten rounds of the following one-arm snatch interval (rest as little as needed between rounds):

15 seconds of one-arm snatches (right arm)
15 seconds of rest
15 seconds of one-arm snatches (left arm)
15 seconds of rest

Remember: When working interval training, the goal is to get in as many reps with good form as possible in the allotted work period. Again, we emphasize *with good form.*

Day 13 — Off

Day 14 — Off

Day 15

Warm-up

5 minutes of unweighted Turkish get-ups
5 minutes of crawling and rolling

Strength training

Power A: 1-2-3-1-2-3-4 ladder
Push A: 1-2-3-1-2-3-4 ladder
Pull A: 1-2-3-1-2-3-4 ladder
Carry A: 1-2-3 ladder

Metabolic conditioning

Two rounds of the following complex (perform each movement on your right side and then immediately on your left before moving to the next exercise):

8 one-arm cleans
5 one-arm racked squats
5 one-arm cleans
3 one-arm racked squats
3 one-arm cleans
2 one-arm racked squats
2 one-arm cleans
1 one-arm racked squat

Day 16

Warm-up

5 minutes of unweighted Turkish get-ups
5 minutes of crawling and rolling

Strength training

Power B: 1-2-3-1-2-3-4 ladder
Push B: 1-2-3-1-2-3-4 ladder
Pull B: 1-2-3-1-2-3-4 ladder
Carry B: 1-2-3 ladder

Metabolic conditioning

5 double kettlebell cleans and 5 double kettlebell front squats on the minute, every minute, for ten minutes

Day 17 — Off

Day 18

Warm-up

5 minutes of unweighted Turkish get-ups
5 minutes of crawling and rolling

Strength training

Hinge A: 1-2-3-1-2-3-4 ladder
Squat A: 1-2-3-1-2-3-4 ladder
Core A: 1-2-3-1-2-3-4 ladder

Metabolic conditioning

5 double cleans and double military presses (that's one double clean between each double press) on the minute, every minute, for 15 minutes

Day 19

Warm-up

5 minutes of unweighted Turkish get-ups
5 minutes of crawling and rolling

Strength training

Hinge B: 1-2-3-1-2-3-4 ladder
Squat B: 1-2-3-1-2-3-4 ladder
Core B: 1-2-3-1-2-3-4 ladder

Metabolic conditioning

20 minutes of interval running (15- to 30-second sprint, 1-minute walk, and then 1-minute jog)

Tip: Interval running is a mix of jogging, sprinting, and walking. The key here is to keep moving but vary the intensity. We recommend the schedule of 1 minute of walking and 1 minute of jogging for every 30 seconds of sprinting. Simply repeat this sequence for whatever amount of time is prescribed.

Day 20 — Off

Day 21 — Off

Day 22

Warm-up

5 minutes of unweighted Turkish get-ups
5 minutes of crawling and rolling

Strength training

Power A: 1-2-3-1-2-3-4 ladder
Push A: 1-2-3-1-2-3-4 ladder
Pull A: 1-2-3-1-2-3-4 ladder
Carry A: 1-2-3 ladder

Metabolic conditioning

Two to three rounds of the following complex:

5 double swings
5 double snatches
5 front squats
5 double military presses
5 double swings

Day 23

Warm-up

5 minutes of unweighted Turkish get-ups
5 minutes of crawling and rolling

Strength training

Power B: 1-2-3-1-2-3-4 ladder
Push B: 1-2-3-1-2-3-4 ladder
Pull B: 1-2-3-1-2-3-4 ladder
Carry B: 1-2-3 ladder

Metabolic conditioning

Four rounds of thruster Tabata intervals (switch sides each working set):

20 seconds of thrusters
10 seconds of rest
20 seconds of thrusters
10 seconds of rest
20 seconds of thrusters

Day 24 — Off

Day 25

Warm-up

5 minutes of unweighted Turkish get-ups
5 minutes of crawling and rolling

Strength training

Hinge A: 1-2-3-4-1-2-3-4 ladder
Squat A: 1-2-3-4-1-2-3-4 ladder
Core A: 1-2-3-4-1-2-3-4 ladder

Metabolic conditioning

Two to three rounds of the following complex (complete entirely on your right side and then immediately on your left):

5 one-arm swings
5 one-arm cleans
5 one-arm snatches
5 one-arm jerks
5 reverse lunges

Day 26

Warm-up

5 minutes of unweighted Turkish get-ups
5 minutes of crawling and rolling

Strength training

Hinge B: 1-2-3-4-1-2-3-4 ladder
Squat B: 1-2-3-4-1-2-3-4 ladder
Core B: 1-2-3-4-1-2-3-4 ladder

Metabolic conditioning

15 minutes of sprints

Day 27 — Off

Day 28 — Off

Day 29

Warm-up

5 minutes of unweighted Turkish get-ups
5 minutes of crawling and rolling

Strength training

Power A: 1-2-3-4-1-2-3-4 ladder
Push A: 1-2-3-4-1-2-3-4 ladder
Pull A: 1-2-3-4-1-2-3-4 ladder
Carry A: 1-2-3-4 ladder

Metabolic conditioning

100 snatches (50 each arm) as quickly as possible with good form

Day 30

Warm-up

5 minutes of unweighted Turkish get-ups
5 minutes of crawling and rolling

Strength training

Power B: 1-2-3-4-1-2-3-4 ladder
Push B: 1-2-3-4-1-2-3-4 ladder
Pull B: 1-2-3-4-1-2-3-4 ladder
Carry B: 1-2-3-4 ladder

Metabolic conditioning

15 minutes of sprints

Day 31 — Off

Day 32

Warm-up

5 minutes of unweighted Turkish get-ups
5 minutes of crawling and rolling

Strength training

Hinge A: 1-2-3-4-1-2-3-4 ladder
Squat A: 1-2-3-4-1-2-3-4 ladder
Core A: 1-2-3-4-1-2-3-4 ladder

Metabolic conditioning

15 minutes of bear crawl sprints

Day 33

Warm-up

5 minutes of unweighted Turkish get-ups
5 minutes of crawling and rolling

Strength training

Hinge B: 1-2-3-4-1-2-3-4 ladder
Squat B: 1-2-3-4-1-2-3-4 ladder
Core B: 1-2-3-4-1-2-3-4 ladder

Metabolic conditioning

Two rounds of the following complex:

8 double cleans
5 double kettlebell front squats
5 double cleans
3 double kettlebell front squats
3 double cleans
2 double kettlebell front squats
2 double cleans
1 double kettlebell front squat

Day 34 — Off

Day 35 — Off

Day 36

Warm-up

5 minutes of unweighted Turkish get-ups
5 minutes of crawling and rolling

Strength training

Power A: 1-2-3-4-1-2-3-4 ladder
Push A: 1-2-3-4-1-2-3-4 ladder
Pull A: 1-2-3-4-1-2-3-4 ladder
Carry A: 1-2-3-4 ladder

Metabolic conditioning

Line up three various weights for two-arm
swings: a light weight, a medium weight,
and a heavy weight. Perform five swings at
each weight. Continue cycling through this
chain for ten minutes.

Day 37

Warm-up

5 minutes of unweighted Turkish get-ups
5 minutes of crawling and rolling

Strength training

Power B: 1-2-3-4-1-2-3-4 ladder
Push B: 1-2-3-4-1-2-3-4 ladder
Pull B: 1-2-3-4-1-2-3-4 ladder
Carry B: 1-2-3-4 ladder

Metabolic conditioning

Perform the following four-round complex:

Round 1:
5 double swings
5 double military presses

Round 2:
5 double swings
5 double cleans
5 double military presses

Round 3:
5 double swings
5 double cleans
5 double snatches
5 double military presses

Round 4:
5 double swings
5 double cleans
5 double snatches
5 double kettlebell front squats
5 double military presses

Day 38 — Off

Day 39

Warm-up

5 minutes of unweighted Turkish get-ups
5 minutes of crawling and rolling

Strength training

Hinge A: 1-2-3-4-1-2-3-4 ladder
Squat A: 1-2-3-4-1-2-3-4 ladder
Core A: 1-2-3-4-1-2-3-4 ladder

Metabolic conditioning

Four rounds of double kettlebell front squat Tabata intervals:

20 seconds of double kettlebell front squats
10 seconds of rest
20 seconds of double kettlebell front squats
10 seconds of rest
20 seconds of double kettlebell front squats
10 seconds of rest

Day 40

Warm-up

5 minutes of unweighted Turkish get-ups
5 minutes of crawling and rolling

Strength training

Hinge B: 1-2-3-4-1-2-3-4 ladder
Squat B: 1-2-3-4-1-2-3-4 ladder
Core B: 1-2-3-4-1-2-3-4 ladder

Metabolic conditioning

20 minutes of interval running

Day 41 — Off

Day 42 — Off

Day 43

Warm-up

5 minutes of unweighted Turkish get-ups
5 minutes of crawling and rolling

Strength training

Power A: 1-2-3-4-1-2-3-4 ladder
Push A: 1-2-3-4-1-2-3-4 ladder
Pull A: 1-2-3-4-1-2-3-4 ladder
Carry A: 1-2-3-4 ladder

Metabolic conditioning

100 one-arm snatches (75 each arm) as
quickly as possible with good form

Tip: A classic test of conditioning and
muscular endurance is the ability to
perform 100 snatches in less than five
minutes while using a 24-kilogram kettlebell (males) or a 16-kilogram kettlebell
(females). Keep this in mind when choosing a weight for this conditioning drill!

Day 44

Warm-up

5 minutes of unweighted Turkish get-ups
5 minutes of crawling and rolling

Strength training

Power B: 1-2-3-4-1-2-3-4 ladder
Push B: 1-2-3-4-1-2-3-4 ladder
Pull B: 1-2-3-4-1-2-3-4 ladder
Carry B: 1-2-3-4 ladder

Metabolic conditioning

15 minutes of bear crawl sprints

Day 45 — Off

Day 46

Warm-up

5 minutes of unweighted Turkish get-ups
5 minutes of crawling and rolling

Strength training

Hinge A: 1-2-3-4-1-2-3-4 ladder
Squat A: 1-2-3-4-1-2-3-4 ladder
Core A: 1-2-3-4-1-2-3-4 ladder

Metabolic conditioning

Three double cleans, two double kettle-
bell front squats, and two double military
presses on the minute, every minute, for ten
minutes

Day 47

Warm-up

5 minutes of unweighted Turkish get-ups
5 minutes of crawling and rolling

Strength training

Hinge B: 1-2-3-4-1-2-3-4 ladder
Squat B: 1-2-3-4-1-2-3-4 ladder
Core B: 1-2-3-4-1-2-3-4 ladder

Metabolic conditioning

Two rounds of the following complex:

10 double swings
10 double snatches
10 double kettlebell front squats
10 double military presses
10 double swings

Day 48 — Off

Day 49 — Off

Day 50

Warm-up

5 minutes of unweighted Turkish get-ups
5 minutes of crawling and rolling

Strength training

Power A: 1-2-3-4-1-2-3-4 ladder
Push A: 1-2-3-4-1-2-3-4 ladder
Pull A: 1-2-3-4-1-2-3-4 ladder
Carry A: 1-2-3-4 ladder

Metabolic conditioning

20 minutes of interval running

Day 51

Warm-up

5 minutes of unweighted Turkish get-ups
5 minutes of crawling and rolling

Strength training

Power B: 1-2-3-4-1-2-3-4 ladder
Push B: 1-2-3-4-1-2-3-4 ladder
Pull B: 1-2-3-4-1-2-3-4 ladder
Carry B: 1-2-3-4 ladder

Metabolic conditioning

One to two rounds of the following complex:

2 double cleans
1 double kettlebell front squat
4 double cleans
2 double kettlebell front squats
6 double cleans
3 double kettlebell front squats
8 double cleans
4 double kettlebell front squats
10 double cleans
5 double kettlebell front squats

Day 52 — Off

Day 53

Warm-up

5 minutes of unweighted Turkish get-ups
5 minutes of crawling and rolling

Strength training

Hinge A: 1-2-3-4-1-2-3-4 ladder
Squat A: 1-2-3-4-1-2-3-4 ladder
Core A: 1-2-3-4-1-2-3-4 ladder

Metabolic conditioning

Five rounds of the following complex (complete entirely on your right side and then immediately on your left):

6 one-arm swings
6 one-arm cleans
6 one-arm snatches
6 one-arm jerks
6 reverse lunges

Day 54

Warm-up

5 minutes of unweighted Turkish get-ups
5 minutes of crawling and rolling

Strength training

Hinge B: 1-2-3-4-1-2-3-4 ladder
Squat B: 1-2-3-4-1-2-3-4 ladder
Core B: 1-2-3-4-1-2-3-4 ladder

Metabolic conditioning

15 minutes of sprints

Day 55 — Off

Day 56 — Off

Day 57

Warm-up

5 minutes of unweighted Turkish get-ups
5 minutes of crawling and rolling

Strength training

Power A: 1-2-3-4-1-2-3-4-5 ladder
Push A: 1-2-3-4-1-2-3-4-5 ladder
Pull A: 1-2-3-4-1-2-3-4-5 ladder
Carry A: 1-2-3-4 ladder

Metabolic conditioning

Perform the following interval sequence of jerks for ten minutes:

15 seconds of one-arm jerks (right arm)
15 seconds of rest
15 seconds of one-arm jerks (left arm)
15 seconds of rest

Day 58

Warm-up

5 minutes of unweighted Turkish get-ups
5 minutes of crawling and rolling

Strength training

Power B: 1-2-3-4-1-2-3-4-5 ladder
Push B: 1-2-3-4-1-2-3-4-5 ladder
Pull B: 1-2-3-4-1-2-3-4-5 ladder
Carry B: 1-2-3-4 ladder

Metabolic conditioning

Four rounds of the following lunge to military press Tabata interval (alternate sides each working set):

20 seconds of lunges to military presses
10 seconds of rest
20 seconds of lunges to military presses
10 seconds of rest
20 seconds of lunges to military presses

Day 59 — Off

Day 60

Warm-up

5 minutes of unweighted Turkish get-ups
5 minutes of crawling and rolling

Strength training

Hinge A: 1-2-3-4-1-2-3-4-5 ladder
Squat A: 1-2-3-4-1-2-3-4-5 ladder
Core A: 1-2-3-4-1-2-3-4-5 ladder

Metabolic conditioning

200 two-arm swings as quickly as possible with good form

Day 61

Warm-up

5 minutes of unweighted Turkish get-ups
5 minutes of crawling and rolling

Strength training

Hinge B: 1-2-3-4-1-2-3-4-5 ladder
Squat B: 1-2-3-4-1-2-3-4-5 ladder
Core B: 1-2-3-4-1-2-3-4-5 ladder

Metabolic conditioning

Ten rounds of the following one-arm snatch interval (rest as little as needed between rounds):

15 seconds of one-arm snatches (right arm)
15 seconds of rest
15 seconds of one-arm snatches (left arm)
15 seconds of rest

Day 62 — Off

Day 63 — Off

Day 64

Warm-up

5 minutes of unweighted Turkish get-ups
5 minutes of crawling and rolling

Strength training

Power A: 1-2-3-4-1-2-3-4-5 ladder
Push A: 1-2-3-4-1-2-3-4-5 ladder
Pull A: 1-2-3-4-1-2-3-4-5 ladder
Carry A: 1-2-3-4

Metabolic conditioning

Five rounds of the following complex:

5 double swings
5 double cleans and military presses (one double clean between each double press)
5 double kettlebell front squats

Day 65

Warm-up

5 minutes of unweighted Turkish get-ups
5 minutes of crawling and rolling

Strength training

Power B: 1-2-3-4-1-2-3-4-5 ladder
Push B: 1-2-3-4-1-2-3-4-5 ladder
Pull B: 1-2-3-4-1-2-3-4-5 ladder
Carry B: 1-2-3-4 ladder

Metabolic conditioning

Ten double snatches on the minute, every minute, for ten minutes

Day 66 — Off

Day 67

Warm-up

5 minutes of unweighted Turkish get-ups
5 minutes of crawling and rolling

Strength training

Hinge A: 1-2-3-4-1-2-3-4-5 ladder
Squat A: 1-2-3-4-1-2-3-4-5 ladder
Core A: 1-2-3-4-1-2-3-4-5 ladder

Metabolic conditioning

15 minutes of sprints

Day 68

Warm-up

5 minutes of unweighted Turkish get-ups
5 minutes of crawling and rolling

Strength training

Hinge B: 1-2-3-4-1-2-3-4-5 ladder
Squat B: 1-2-3-4-1-2-3-4-5 ladder
Core B: 1-2-3-4-1-2-3-4-5 ladder

Metabolic conditioning

Five rounds of the following complex:

1 double clean
3 double military presses
2 front squats
10 double swings

Day 69 — Off

Day 70 — Off

Day 71

Warm-up

5 minutes of unweighted Turkish get-ups
5 minutes of crawling and rolling

Strength training

Power A: 1-2-3-4-1-2-3-4-5 ladder
Push A: 1-2-3-4-1-2-3-4-5 ladder
Pull A: 1-2-3-4-1-2-3-4-5 ladder
Carry A: 1-2-3-4 ladder

Metabolic conditioning

15 minutes of bear crawl sprints

Day 72

Warm-up

5 minutes of unweighted Turkish get-ups
5 minutes of crawling and rolling

Strength training

Power B: 1-2-3-4-1-2-3-4-5 ladder
Push B: 1-2-3-4-1-2-3-4-5 ladder
Pull B: 1-2-3-4-1-2-3-4-5 ladder
Carry B: 1-2-3-4 ladder

Metabolic conditioning

Two rounds of the following complex:

15 double swings
15 double snatches
15 double kettlebell front squats
15 double military presses
15 push-ups

Day 73 — Off

Day 74

Warm-up

5 minutes of unweighted Turkish get-ups
5 minutes of crawling and rolling

Strength training

Hinge A: 1-2-3-4-1-2-3-4-5 ladder
Squat A: 1-2-3-4-1-2-3-4-5 ladder
Core A: 1-2-3-4-1-2-3-4-5 ladder

Metabolic conditioning

20 minutes of interval running

Day 75

Warm-up

5 minutes of unweighted Turkish get-ups
5 minutes of crawling and rolling

Strength training

Hinge B: 1-2-3-4-1-2-3-4-5 ladder
Squat B: 1-2-3-4-1-2-3-4-5 ladder
Core B: 1-2-3-4-1-2-3-4-5 ladder

Metabolic conditioning

Five rounds of the following complex
(complete entirely on your right side and
then immediately on your left):

5 one-arm swings
5 one-arm cleans
5 one-arm snatches
5 racked squats
5 push presses
5 reverse lunges

Day 76 — Off

Day 77 — Off

Day 78

Warm-up

5 minutes of unweighted Turkish get-ups
5 minutes of crawling and rolling

Strength training

Power A: 1-2-3-4-5-1-2-3-4-5 ladder
Push A: 1-2-3-4-5-1-2-3-4-5 ladder
Pull A: 1-2-3-4-5-1-2-3-4-5 ladder
Carry A: 1-2-3-4 ladder

Metabolic conditioning

150 one-arm snatches (75 each arm) as quickly as possible with good form

Day 79

Warm-up

5 minutes of unweighted Turkish get-ups
5 minutes of crawling and rolling

Strength training

Power B: 1-2-3-4-5-1-2-3-4-5 ladder
Push B: 1-2-3-4-5-1-2-3-4-5 ladder
Pull B: 1-2-3-4-5-1-2-3-4-5 ladder
Carry B: 1-2-3-4 ladder

Metabolic conditioning

Two rounds of the following complex:

15 double swings
15 double snatches
15 double kettlebell front squats
15 double military presses
15 push-ups

Day 80 — Off

Day 81

Warm-up

5 minutes of unweighted Turkish get-ups
5 minutes of crawling and rolling

Strength training

Hinge A: 1-2-3-4-5-1-2-3-4-5 ladder
Squat A: 1-2-3-4-5-1-2-3-4-5 ladder
Core A: 1-2-3-4-5-1-2-3-4-5 ladder

Metabolic conditioning

20 minutes of interval running

Day 82

Warm-up

5 minutes of unweighted Turkish get-ups
5 minutes of crawling and rolling

Strength training

Hinge B: 1-2-3-4-5-1-2-3-4-5 ladder
Squat B: 1-2-3-4-5-1-2-3-4-5 ladder
Core B: 1-2-3-4-5-1-2-3-4-5 ladder

Metabolic conditioning

15 minutes of bear crawl sprints

Day 83 — Off

Day 84 — Off

Day 85

Warm-up

5 minutes of unweighted Turkish get-ups
5 minutes of crawling and rolling

Strength training

Power A: 1-2-3-4-5-1-2-3-4-5 ladder
Push A: 1-2-3-4-5-1-2-3-4-5 ladder
Pull A: 1-2-3-4-5-1-2-3-4-5 ladder
Carry A: 1-2-3-4 ladder

Metabolic conditioning

Four rounds of the following two-arm swing Tabata interval:

20 seconds of two-arm swings
10 seconds of rest
20 seconds of two-arm swings
10 seconds of rest
20 seconds of two-arm swings

Day 86

Warm-up

5 minutes of unweighted Turkish get-ups
5 minutes of crawling and rolling

Strength training

Power B: 1-2-3-4-5-1-2-3-4-5 ladder
Push B: 1-2-3-4-5-1-2-3-4-5 ladder
Pull B: 1-2-3-4-5-1-2-3-4-5 ladder
Carry B: 1-2-3-4 ladder

Metabolic conditioning

Two to three rounds of the following complex (perform entirely on your right side and then immediately on your left):

5 one-arm swings
5 one-arm cleans and military presses (one clean between each press)
5 one-arm push presses
5 reverse lunges
5 single-leg dead lifts

Day 87 — Off

Day 88

Warm-up

5 minutes of unweighted Turkish get-ups
5 minutes of crawling and rolling

Strength training

Hinge A: 1-2-3-4-5-1-2-3-4-5 ladder
Squat A: 1-2-3-4-5-1-2-3-4-5 ladder
Core A: 1-2-3-4-5-1-2-3-4-5 ladder

Metabolic conditioning

15 minutes of sprints

Day 89

Warm-up

5 minutes of unweighted Turkish get-ups
5 minutes of crawling and rolling

Strength training

Hinge B: 1-2-3-4-5-1-2-3-4-5 ladder
Squat B: 1-2-3-4-5-1-2-3-4-5 ladder
Core B: 1-2-3-4-5-1-2-3-4-5 ladder

Metabolic conditioning

Two to three rounds of the following complex:

15 double swings
15 double snatches
15 double cleans and military presses (one double clean between each double press)
15 front squats
15 push-ups

Day 90 — Off and Done!

Don't forget to take your final progress pictures!

Chapter 14

Specialized Paleo Fitness Programs

* * *

* * *

*T*his chapter is dedicated to athletes. Here, we show you how to adjust the primal exercise programs while in and out of season.

All the Paleo fitness principles we discuss in Chapter 2, such as focusing on strength, practicing diaphragmatic breathing, and moving on a daily basis, hold true for athletes. For example, most athletes need to spend more time on low-rep, high-quality strength training than anything else. But too many athletes spend too much time in the weight room, violating the minimalism principle. Instead, athletes should spend the least amount of time needed in the weight room because the majority of their time is better invested in practicing their specific sport skills.

Most athletes work on things without knowing why they're working on them or even stopping to think whether they should be working on them. The two most common offenders are the bench press and the back squat. No doubt these two lifts can produce results, but you must ask yourself whether these results are going to make you a better athlete.

Any exercise in an athletic training program should exhibit a sufficient reason for being there. As elite strength coach Jim Ferris says, "The purpose of training is to train with purpose." So if you can reasonably justify bench pressing in your strength-training routine (most people can't) and also justify that it's better than any possible alternative, then include it. If you can't, scrap it.

We're not here to say that any one exercise is wrong for athletes. Every athlete is different and has unique strengths and weaknesses. And an exercise that may be appropriate for one athlete may be inappropriate for another, even though they may be in the same sport.

In this chapter, we give you a set of guidelines to help you make an informed decision on how to best incorporate Paleo fitness into your athletic training program. From building muscle to staying fit in your older years, from improving in your athletic sport-specific skills to exercising while pregnant, we give you the tools you need to make the Paleo fitness program your own. And in making it your own, it will be reasonable, sustainable, and personalized — and, therefore, more likely to work successfully for you.

Training, Practice, and the Paleo Athlete

Training is training. Practice is practice. There is a difference.

In training, athletes work in a controlled environment to improve on their physical weaknesses, or at least that's how it should be. In practice, athletes work on improving their specific sports skills.

In training, athletes work on improving their general physical preparedness — strength, conditioning, mobility, stability, agility, and so on. This baseline competency gives athletes a small advantage. In practice, athletes work on improving their sport-specific preparedness — the skills that pertain particularly to their sport. Their proficiency here gives them a large advantage.

So, for example, the best basketball players aren't necessarily the ones who can squat the most weight; they're the ones who can play the best basketball. To forget this distinction is a common error, and the result is too much time spent on training and too little time spent on practice.

When athletes overemphasize training, the drawbacks are both plain and severe. For one, they have less time to dedicate to their specific skill development, so it suffers in quantity. And they have less nerve energy to allot to their sport-specific training, so it suffers in quality.

As an athlete, you should use training to "fill in the gaps," as renowned strength and conditioning coach Dan John would say. In other words, no athlete is ever a complete athlete, but the purpose of your training should be to bring you closer to completion.

If you lack strength — a common enough gap — then the major function of your training should be to fill that gap. If you suffer from movement dysfunction — also a common gap — then your training should serve to remedy that.

A good athletic training program is the direct result of an accurate inference from a sound observation. In other words, when you take the time to identify the gaps (a sound observation) and intelligently identify the cause of those gaps (an accurate inference), then, and only then, can you prescribe an appropriate training regimen.

In the following sections, we explore what makes an athlete who follows the Paleo plan different and also explain the benefits of a primal fitness program.

What makes the Paleo athlete different

The Paleo athlete is one who understands and masters primal movement patterns, cultivates strength, and ultimately has a better chance of staying fit, strong, and healthy throughout his life. You don't have to be "an athlete" in the strictest sense of the word, but in adhering to a Paleo exercise regimen, such as the ones outlined in this book, you will become an athlete. A Paleo athlete.

Here are a few other characteristics of the Paleo athlete:

- Adheres to a minimalistic approach to training
- Takes the time to identify gaps, acknowledges the causes, and then diligently pursues corrections
- Doesn't squat for the sake of squatting, bench for the sake of benching, or curl for the sake of curling
- Understands why he's doing what he's doing and, if asked, can clearly explain it to you

The Paleo athlete further understands that the majority of time should be spent on practice. And the amount of time he spends in the weight room is delicately balanced somewhere between as long as he has to and as little as he needs to.

The Paleo athlete doesn't waste time on *superfluous activities* — any activity that doesn't directly benefit the athlete in a sensible way — because he understands that energy is limited and must be thoughtfully invested into the activities that are going to offer him the greatest expected return.

The benefits of a primal approach to athletic development

Our approach to athletic development — what we've affectionately dubbed *the primal approach* because it shares so many similarities to the principles of Paleo fitness — is a minimalistic approach. Compared to the conventional approach, the benefits are many, including the following:

- ✔ Training is largely focused on improving weaknesses, whatever they may be.

- ✔ Training is used to enhance practice, never detract from it.

- ✔ Emphasis is more on movement quality and a reduced risk of injury.

- ✔ Precious nerve energy isn't wasted on frivolous activities and is thus saved for more important sport-specific skill work.

- ✔ It is flexible and may be molded around the capabilities of the athlete.

The Cave Man Athlete Program

In general, most athletes will profit from following the 90-Day Primal Body Transformation program (see Chapter 13), with just a few minor tweaks depending on the sport, the athlete, and the season. Most of these tweaks will be ways of reduction — that is, taking away from the program rather than adding to it — to ensure that the athlete isn't wasting more energy on her strength and conditioning program than necessary.

In the following sections, we give you a brief overview of how to follow the primal exercise program both in season and off-season.

Staying strong in season

In season, you should follow the 90-day program but switch to a three-day split. The following schedule works well for most athletes:

- ✔ Day 1: On
- ✔ Day 2: Off
- ✔ Day 3: On
- ✔ Day 4: Off

✔ Day 5: On

✔ Day 6: Off

✔ Day 7: Off

Naturally, with the additional rest days, the program stretches beyond 90 days, but that doesn't matter because you'll follow the program only for as long as you're in season with your sport. You'll also cut your metabolic conditioning work down to one to two days per week. Start with one day a week, and if your conditioning still lags after a couple weeks, add in another day. Metabolic conditioning drains the nervous system, and too much will make your sport performance suffer.

You get most of your conditioning from the actual sport practice itself. You should use metabolic conditioning only as a supplement to that conditioning. Be sure to apply it judiciously.

Filling in the gaps during the off-season

The off-season is best spent addressing specific weaknesses and imbalances, whatever they may be. This is your chance to "fill in the gaps."

Really, the off-season is where you "swallow the frog first," so to speak — or do the things you know you really need to do but don't particularly like to do. If you have mobility issues, then you need to work on mobility. If you're imbalanced between upper- and lower-body strength, then the off-season is the time to correct that.

To figure out what to do during the off-season, you may need to seek out a qualified coach. In fact, we recommend you do so. Because each individual's needs are different, we can't prescribe a one-size-fits-all program for the off-season to address these weaknesses, but a coach can help you pinpoint your specific needs and help you work on them.

Building Paleo Muscle: The Primal Method for Muscle Mass

Our 90-day program isn't a bulking program, but what if you want a bulking program? Is there a primal approach to putting on lean muscle mass?

The answer is yes. Although you'll gain a considerable amount of lean, functional muscle mass from the 90-day program, that is only a consequence of chasing strength, not a direct pursuit. In this section, we roll out a program specifically designed for putting on as much lean muscle mass as possible in a safe and efficient manner. We call it the Paleo Muscle Program. In the following sections, we outline this program, starting with food and then moving on to the exercises and a sample workout.

Food = muscle

Before beginning the Paleo Muscle Program, you must first understand that your ability to put on muscle is ultimately reduced to your ability to eat for muscle. If you don't eat enough while following this program, you may actually lose weight. However, we're not giving you an excuse to eat like a pig. Keep your eating clean and primal; just eat more and more often. At the end of the day, you putting on weight will still be the direct result of you taking in more calories than you're putting out — this program simply primes the system to use those calories to manufacture lean muscle mass rather than fat.

For more information on what foods to eat (and which ones to avoid), check out Part IV of this book, where we discuss how the Paleo diet can help you optimize your Paleo fitness routine.

The exercises and routines

The Paleo Muscle Program is tough, and it includes only four exercises: the dead lift, the double clean and military press (which is a double kettlebell clean followed immediately by a double kettlebell military press), the dip, and the front squat. (**Note:** Although we prefer the dip, especially a weighted dip, you may substitute with the bench press.)

Muscular hypertrophy — the increase in size of skeletal muscle — is largely a function of finding the appropriate amounts of tension and the right amount of time spent under that tension. In other words, to facilitate muscle growth, or more specifically, as much muscle growth as possible, you have to employ just the right amount of weight and just the right amount of time under that weight.

Bodybuilders, whose purpose is to maximize hypertrophy, typically employ a range of 8 to 12 reps and may work anywhere between three to five sets per muscle group. But because this is a primal exercise book, and because we choose not to train any particular muscle group in isolation but rather the body as a whole, we take a slightly different approach to muscle.

Using only these four big movements, we employ a set-and-rep scheme of ten sets by five repetitions, with only 60 to 120 seconds of rest between each set. With a quick calculation, that's a total of 50 reps. This scheme provides an adequate amount of volume (total work performed), density (work performed within a certain time parameter), and intensity (weight moved) to trigger muscle growth while still training the big, compound, strength-building movements.

In Table 14-1, we outline an example of the Paleo Muscle Program workout.

Table 14-1	Paleo Muscle Program Workout Sample		
Day	*Exercise*	*Number of Reps*	*Number of Sets*
Monday	Double clean and military press	5	10
	Dead lift	5	10
Tuesday	Weighted dip	5	10
	Front squat	5	10
Wednesday	Off		
Thursday	Double clean and military press	5	10
	Dead lift	5	10
Friday	Weighted dip	5	10
	Front squat	5	10
Saturday	Off		
Sunday	Off		

Addressing the Fitness Needs of the Young, the Old, and the Expecting

As you may already realize, the question isn't *if* Paleo fitness is for you but *how* Paleo fitness is for you. In this section, we address how to make Paleo fitness more accessible throughout various phases of life — whether you're a young adult just starting a fitness routine, an older adult trying to figure out how to move with quality, or an expectant mother wanting to keep fit during your pregnancy.

No matter what phase of life you're in, be sure to secure your doctor's approval before beginning an exercise program.

Building a foundation: Paleo fitness for the young adult

People are malleable, and the young adult is especially so. Although people are never not malleable, throughout the years, they begin to stiffen up quite a bit. Breaking habits and establishing new ones become more difficult.

So for the young adult (anyone between 14 and 24 years old), the most important function of Paleo fitness — which is arguably the most important function of Paleo fitness in general — is to get into the habit of moving well. How you learn to move now is how you'll move later on.

And if you're wondering whether you should lift weights, the answer is yes. The research is clear: Weight training benefits the young adult in much the same way as it benefits everyone else.

Here are a few benefits of weight training:

- ✔ Builds bone strength
- ✔ Builds lean muscle
- ✔ Builds motor control
- ✔ Builds strength, power, and endurance
- ✔ Decreases body fat (when in conjunction with a healthy diet)
- ✔ Increases confidence

As a young adult, your first goal should be to master all the basic and intermediary movements found throughout Part II of this book. You'll profit enormously from practicing all these movements in a low-rep, high-quality manner. You should practice them the same way you'd practice the piano — slowly at first, a highly focused effort with intensive concentration and attention to detail.

But before even that, you should spend as much time as necessary to master the following movements:

- ✔ The **kettlebell swing** (or just "swing") is high velocity but low impact, meaning it's great for building power and endurance, but it's still friendly on the joints. For step-by-step instructions on how to perform the swing, see Chapter 5.

✔ The **goblet squat** loosens the hips while strengthening the legs and the core. For step-by-step instructions on how to perform the goblet squat, see Chapter 5.

✔ The **Turkish get-up** is one of the best tools to teach young adults how to move well. It utilizes each of the major muscle groups in the body, while honing skills, such as balance and *proprioception* — your awareness of self or sense of relative position in space. For step-by-step instructions on how to perform the Turkish get-up, see Chapter 3.

Really, a two- to three-day-a-week exercise program is plenty for most young adults. And each training session should last between 15 and 20 minutes, divided up evenly between these three movements.

As for selecting a weight, choose one that's challenging but manageable. For the most part, a 10- to 35-pound weight is a good starting point for any of these three exercises.

From there, you should follow the same path as everyone else and enter into the 21-Day Primal Quick Start program (see Chapter 12). If, after the 21-day program, you feel like you have a solid understanding of the movements as well as an adequate strength and conditioning base, you may then proceed on to the 90-Day Primal Body Transformation program (see Chapter 13).

Adjusting Paleo fitness for boomers and seniors

Just like young adults, most boomers and seniors need to (re)discover how to move well because improving movement quality greatly reduces risk of injury. And so you may find it slightly ironic that the boomer and senior program closely mimics the young adult program.

After you're cleared by your doctor, your program will be to focus on mastering the three following movements (refer to the previous section for a description and Chapters 3 and 5 for details):

✔ The swing

✔ The goblet squat

✔ The Turkish get-up

Unable to do a full Turkish get-up due to prior injuries or movement restrictions? No worries! You can always just work parts of the get-up rather than the whole. Almost everyone can do and benefit from the first stage of the get-up (the roll).

When you're proficient in all three of these movements, you may then proceed on to the 21-Day Primal Quick Start program (Chapter 12). But only if you want to! You can very well just continue on with these three movements for, well, indefinitely — yep, they're that good!

Finally, after the 21-Day Quick Start, if all is well and good, even boomers and seniors may move on to the full 90-Day Primal Body Transformation program (Chapter 13), with just a few minor adjustments. The first is to cut the training down to only two to three days a week. As people age, it takes longer to recover. Subtracting work and adding in additional rest days is often necessary for the more mature among us.

Exercising when you're expecting

First off, congratulations! Pregnancy is a beautiful, miraculous part of life. It can also be incredibly challenging. But one thing you can do to make the whole process easier is to keep fit! And evidence now shows that exercising while pregnant benefits not only the mom but also the baby. Here, we outline the benefits of keeping fit while pregnant and also introduce you to the movements you can continue throughout your pregnancy.

Naturally, if you're pregnant, consult with your doctor before beginning any exercise program. Take this book to your doctor and discuss the program with him or her. Let it be known that with this program you'll be lifting weights and your heart rate will be elevated. It's essential that you get your doctor's clearance before starting this, or any other, program.

The benefits of exercising while pregnant

Being pregnant is an invalid excuse to not exercise. Even if you've never exercised before pregnancy, most doctors now agree that starting an exercise program is not only safe but also highly beneficial. Prenatal exercise boosts energy, relieve aches and pains, and increases confidence. What's more is that those who exercise regularly throughout pregnancy often report a smoother labor.

Here are some of the other potential benefits of prenatal exercise:

✔ Better sleep
✔ Increased vitality

  ✔ Fewer odds of gestational diabetes

  ✔ Shorter labor

  ✔ Better birth outcomes

  ✔ Quicker postpartum recovery

Paleo exercises during pregnancy

What exercises should a mom-to-be do? Well, swings, goblet squats, and Turkish get-ups, of course — just like anyone else (see the earlier section "Building a foundation: Paleo fitness for the young adult" for descriptions on these movements). These movements will help prep the body for labor in a unique way. For example, they all serve to strengthen the abdominal wall and the pelvic floor (similar to kegels).

Never do an exercise you're uncomfortable with or unsure about when expecting. The pregnant body releases a hormone (relaxin) to lubricate the joints and prepare the body for labor. Although increased suppleness is desired for delivery, it may increase your risk of injury if you're inexperienced. So when starting out, take your time, keep it light, and stick to what you're comfortable with.

Start out by "practicing" these movements and be sure to master the dead lift before going into the two-arm swing. Take your time and work only a few repetitions at any one time. After you feel good with these three movements, you may want to add in planks (see Figure 14-1), lunges, presses, goblet squats (see Figure 14-2), and other movements.

Figure 14-1:
Planks keep your core strong and help you fight off back pain throughout pregnancy.

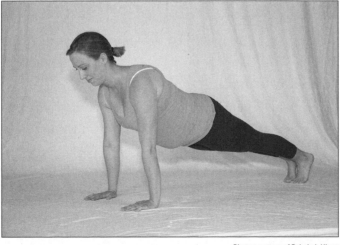

Photo courtesy of Rebekah Ulmer

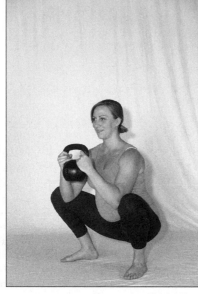

Figure 14-2:
The goblet
squat is a
wonder-
ful way to
prepare the
body for
delivery.

Photo courtesy of Rebekah Ulmer

Following are a few beginner pregnancy workouts to try (see Chapters 3, 5, and 7 for the full steps on these movements):

✔ **Pregnancy Workout 1:**

• Warm-up: 5 minutes of unweighted Turkish get-ups

• Exercise 1: Five 5-rep sets of goblet squats

• Exercise 2: Five 10-rep sets of two-arm swings

• Exercise 3: Three 30-second sets of four-point planks

✔ **Pregnancy Workout 2:**

• Warm-up: 5 minutes of unweighted Turkish get-ups

• Exercise 1: Three 5-rep sets of cleans and presses (five reps each side)

• Exercise 2: Three 5-rep sets of alternating lunges (five reps each side)

• Exercise 3: Five 10-rep sets of two-arm swings

• Exercise 4: Three 30-second sets of four-point planks

✔ **Pregnancy Workout 3:**

- Warm-up: 5 minutes of unweighted Turkish get-ups

- Exercise 1: Five 10-rep sets of one-arm swings (ten reps each side)

- Exercise 2: Five 5-rep sets of goblet squats

- Exercise 3: Three 5-rep sets of single-leg dead lifts (five reps each leg)

- Exercise 4: Three 30-second sets of four-point planks

From here, and with your doctor's approval, you may move on to the 21-Day Primal Quick Start program (Chapter 12), making any adjustments as needed.

We don't recommend the full 90-Day Primal Body Transformation program (from Chapter 13) as a prenatal exercise program because of its relatively high intensity. Save that program for part of your postnatal recovery plan!

Part IV
Paleo Nutrition

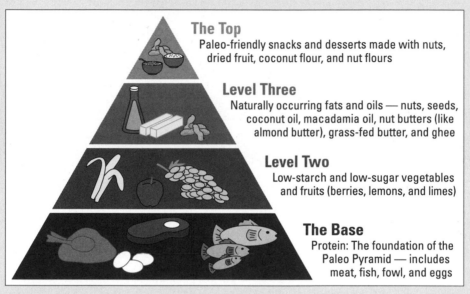

The Top
Paleo-friendly snacks and desserts made with nuts, dried fruit, coconut flour, and nut flours

Level Three
Naturally occurring fats and oils — nuts, seeds, coconut oil, macadamia oil, nut butters (like almond butter), grass-fed butter, and ghee

Level Two
Low-starch and low-sugar vegetables and fruits (berries, lemons, and limes)

The Base
Protein: The foundation of the Paleo Pyramid — includes meat, fish, fowl, and eggs

Illustration by Wiley, Composition Services Graphics

Choosing the right foods can help you perform better when exercising. Check out www.dummies.com/extras/paleoworkouts for information on the benefits of including healthy fats in your diet.

In this part . . .

- ✔ Find out which foods you should chuck from your freezer, refrigerator, pantry, and life to realize optimal health on the Paleo diet.

- ✔ Replace common everyday foods with gluten-free, dairy-free, and nutrient-dense Paleo foods.

- ✔ Recognize the benefits of the Paleo diet for athletes of all kinds, from the weekend warrior to the elite endurance athlete.

- ✔ Take Paleo living beyond nutrition and exercise with relaxation, quality sleep, good sun exposure, and clean water.

Chapter 15

Paleo Foods

· ·

· ·

*Y*our body is designed to eat certain foods. The closer you stick to these foods, the better you'll look and feel. Much of the food available today may seem like common, everyday nutritional options, but from an *evolutionary* standpoint, they're really quite new. Your body has a hard time running efficiently or digesting these foods. Discovering Paleo foods and how to transform your kitchen into a place that moves your body toward health is truly the foundation for high performance.

You can make eating healthy really simple. It doesn't have to be over-the-top or difficult, and you don't have to use hard-to-find or unusual ingredients. Eating Paleo is about eating simple, back-to-nature foods put together in a simple way, without making you feel like you're missing out or, worse yet, dieting.

If you're a newcomer to the kitchen, don't be intimidated. These foods are packed with nutrition and easy to work with. We know that if it's not easy, you won't go for it! You have a busy life, and we want to make your life as easy and healthy as possible, certainly not more overwhelming or exhausting.

Bottom line: It's time to get your fanny in the kitchen and start preparing the foods you were designed to eat. In this chapter, we show you what foods will get you leaner, stronger, and healthier and which ones you can (and should) do without. We also clue you in to the types of food and the times best suited for pre- and post-workout meals to give you a boost in performance.

Choosing the Right Foods for the Paleo Lifestyle

We love Paleo foods because we know that they help you look and feel your best and definitely help you perform your best. Paleo foods are lean proteins, fish and seafood, vegetables, small amounts of fruits, nuts, and seeds, and little to no sugars. The closer you stick to these foods, the healthier you'll be. In the following sections, we explain what foods you should avoid and what Paleo foods you want to stock in your fridge, freezer, and pantry.

Eliminating foods from your diet

If you really want to eat Paleo, you can't have a lot of other foods hanging around. To be really committed, your best bet is to go through your kitchen, inventory what you have, and remove all the foods that aren't part of the Paleo food plan.

Cleaning out your kitchen makes everything easier. It's no different from cleaning out your closet. Honestly, after you clean out your closet, don't you instantly feel lighter and more inspired? Most of all, when you clean out your kitchen, you get clarity. You know exactly what you have to work with, and you don't have a bunch of clutter tugging at you, making your transition to Paleo even more difficult.

When you clean out your kitchen of the non-Paleo foods and restock with nutrient-rich Paleo goodness, you're less tempted to buy foods that aren't part of your new eating habits. But before you restock with all the amazing foods we recommend, you have to get in the game. You have to clean out your kitchen and make way for eating Paleo.

And with that, here are some foods you want to cleanse from your kitchen once and for all:

- All foods with flour, including breads, pasta, crackers, chips, and cookies
- All foods with grains and whole grains, including wheat, barley, rye, oats, spelt, corn, and quinoa
- Refined processed fats, such as canola (rapeseed), soybean, grape seed, sunflower, safflower, corn, margarine, vegetable, and peanut oils
- Hydrogenated or partially hydrogenated oils (cookies, snack foods, and buttery spreads)
- All foods with artificial sweeteners, such as acesulfame-K (Sweet One), aspartame (Equal and NutraSweet), saccharin (Sweet'N Low), and sucralose (Splenda)

✔ High-fructose corn syrup and all other sugars except for raw honey, pure maple syrup, dark chocolate, and cocoa powder

✔ Packaged processed foods like microwavable meals or food bars (Check all processed foods carefully because most have additives and gluten.)

✔ All soy *frankenfoods* — processed foods made to look like a certain food product but are really made from wheat, such as vegetarian burgers, hot dogs, and chicken nuggets

Stocking your fridge with Paleo foods

When you switch to eating Paleo, you want to stock your fridge with meats, fish, and produce. These foods become your baseline for fuel, or energy. Your body is designed to eat these foods, and these foods will make you leaner, stronger, and healthier.

Proteins

When you can, your best protein options are always meat from organic, pasture-raised, antibiotic-free sources. If buying organic isn't in the budget, don't let it stress you out. Buying the leanest cuts you can find, removing the skin on poultry and the excess fat on red meat before cooking, and removing and draining excess fat after cooking is a great strategy to making conventional meats as healthy as possible.

When it comes to pork, organ meats, and deli meats, we say if you can't get an organic source to avoid the toxins, opt for a different protein source. Here's a list of Paleo-approved proteins:

✔ Beef

✔ Eggs

✔ Fish and seafood

✔ Game meats

✔ Lamb

✔ Organic, nitrite- and gluten-free deli meats and sausages

✔ Organic, pasture-raised organ meats (liver, kidney, and heart)

✔ Pork

✔ Poultry

When buying eggs, organic and pastured-raised are best. Labels or cartons that read *vegetarian fed* and *natural* don't tell you the quality of the eggs.

Vegetables

Veggies provide a great source of energy and tons of nutrition and fiber. Getting energy naturally with these vegetables makes your body run better than any modern-day carbohydrates can do. Try to eat two different vegetables with a meal, choosing from any in the following list:

- Artichoke
- Arugula
- Asparagus
- Beets
- Bell peppers
- Bok choy
- Broccoli
- Brussels sprouts
- Cabbage
- Carrots
- Cassava
- Cauliflower
- Celery
- Chile peppers
- Cucumber
- Eggplant
- Endive
- Escarole
- Garlic
- Green beans
- Greens: beet, collard, mustard, and turnip
- Kale
- Kohlrabi

- Leeks
- Lettuces
- Mushrooms
- Nori (seaweed)
- Okra
- Onion
- Parsnip
- Plantain
- Pumpkin
- Radish
- Rutabaga
- Shallots
- Snow peas
- Spaghetti squash
- Spinach
- Sugar snap peas
- Summer squash
- Sweet potatoes/yams
- Taro root
- Tomatillos
- Tomatoes
- Turnips
- Winter squash: butternut and acorn

Several veggies — acorn squash, beets, butternut squash, carrots, cassava, kohlrabi, onion, parsnip, plantain, pumpkin, rutabaga, spaghetti squash, summer squash, sweet potatoes/yams, taro root, and turnips — also qualify as *dense carbohydrates* because they're more "starchy." These veggies are perfect to include in any post-workout meal because they restore your muscles with what they need for recovery — a far better choice than a bagel or a bowl of pasta! For some tasty, simple recipes using these veggies, check out *Paleo Cookbook For Dummies* (Wiley).

Fruits

Eating delicious and juicy fruits are a great way to satisfy your sweet tooth, or you can use fruits in cooking as a natural sweetener. Just don't let fruits push vegetables off your plate! You want to eat fruit in moderation: Two small pieces a day, or a handful of berries twice a day should do it. Also, limit your consumption of dried fruit; it's easy to overeat, and it lacks the nutrition of fresh fruits, while concentrating the sugars. Here are some great fruits to choose from:

- Apple
- Apricot
- Banana
- Berries: blackberries, blueberries, cranberries, raspberries, and strawberries
- Cantaloupe
- Cherries
- Date
- Fig
- Grapefruit
- Grapes
- Honeydew
- Kiwi
- Kumquat

- Lemon
- Lime
- Lychee
- Mango
- Nectarine
- Oranges: mandarin, clementine, and tangerine
- Papaya
- Peach
- Pear
- Pineapple
- Plum
- Pomegranate
- Watermelon

Condiments

Condiments without added flours, sugars, or poor-quality oils in them are tough to find. Mustard is a pretty safe bet; just be sure to check the label for gluten. For ketchup, dressings, and dipping sauces, we suggest you grab a copy of *Paleo Cookbook For Dummies* (Wiley), where you'll find great recipes that are easy to make and super delicious.

Storing Paleo-approved foods in your freezer

You freezer may have an entirely different look to it after getting rid of the frozen pre-made meals, pizzas, waffles, or microwave meals. These foods are definitely not Paleo! What you'll see in your freezer from now on is really pretty basic and includes the following:

- ✔ Fruits
- ✔ Lean meats and fish
- ✔ Packaged Paleo meals that you prepared and froze yourself
- ✔ Vegetables

Eating frozen fruits and vegetables are second-best to eating seasonal local produce, because they're flash frozen and maintain much of their nutrients in this process. We also love the idea of pre-making Paleo meals for the week, or *batch cooking,* because preparing food ahead of time actually saves you time and money in the long run; it also keeps you from getting caught off guard. Being hungry and having no food ready to go may just have you diving head-first into a bowl of ice cream. And that's something you don't want to do as you transition to Paleo.

Stowing Paleo goods in your pantry

Pantry foods can make a big difference. If you're not careful, you can easily pack your pantry full of foods you find in the middle of the grocery store — often processed, packaged foods. When shopping for pantry items, reading labels is important. Make sure you're not picking a product with added sugars (real or artificial), soy, gluten, or chemical preservatives.

To help you get started with the perfect pantry items, here are some great Paleo-approved pantry finds:

- ✔ Almond meal (instead of flour)
- ✔ Arrowroot powder (substitute for flour and cornstarch and use as thickener)
- ✔ Artichoke hearts
- ✔ Beef jerky (gluten- and soy-free)
- ✔ Broth: chicken, beef, and vegetable
- ✔ Canned chilies

- ✔ Coconut aminos (instead of soy sauce)

- ✔ Canned fish: tuna, salmon, and sardines

- ✔ Canned tomatoes, tomato paste, and tomato sauce

- ✔ Coconut flour (instead of flour)

- ✔ Fish sauce (Red Boat brand is good)

- ✔ Hot sauce

- ✔ Salsa

Along with these pantry staples, fats nourish every structure and function of the body, including your very important brain. Fats also help you absorb nutrients more efficiently and keep you feeling full.

Choose from any of the following fats for your Paleo pantry and see our suggestions for substituting the ones you pitched from your pre-Paleo kitchen:

- ✔ Coconut: butter, fresh, flakes, and milk

- ✔ Nuts and nut butters: almonds, Brazil nuts, cashews, chestnuts, hazelnuts, macadamia nuts, pecans, pistachios, and walnuts

- ✔ Oils: macadamia, avocado, coconut, olive, and walnut

- ✔ Olives: black, green, pimento (watch the label to make sure they're not cured in high amounts of sodium)

- ✔ Seeds: pumpkin, sesame, sunflower, pine nuts

Fueling Your Body for Maximum Performance

The goal for the Paleo athlete is to optimize performance and improve recovery. The Paleo diet provides the foods you need for high performance and recovery in spades.

Why eating lean proteins, vegetables, fruits, healthy fats, nuts, and seeds are great fuel for performance is no secret: These foods have massive *nutrient density* — a high number of nutrition for the calories the food contains — which helps you perform your best and recover quickly.

In the following sections, we outline what makes Paleo foods so effective for athletic performance and also tell you the best foods to eat before and after a workout.

Packing a (nutritional) punch with Paleo

This question comes up often: "Will Paleo foods provide me with the nutrition I need for performance?" The answer is, absolutely! In fact, Paleo foods provide you with some of the most valuable resources to help you perform your best. And Paleo foods can give you your competitive edge. For example, here are three nutritional bonuses you gain from putting Paleo foods into play:

- ✔ **Aminos to the rescue:** The lean meat and fish provide you with a healthy dose of *branched-chain amino acids* (BCAAs). BCAAs are different from other amino acids that together make up protein because they help build and repair muscle. BCAAs are perfect for performance athletes who are constantly breaking down, building, and repairing tissue.

- ✔ **Nutrients times 10:** All the vitamins, minerals, antioxidants, phytochemicals, and B vitamins found in Paleo-approved foods make them super-foods for fueling, repairing, and recovering.

- ✔ **Fit fuel:** The fuel athletes love is in the form of *glycogen,* which is essential particularly for intense exercise. This fuel doesn't come from protein or fat but in the form of Paleo-approved starches (or dense carbohydrates). Great sources are yams, pumpkin, squash, jicama, carrots, beets, and bananas.

When you eat Paleo, all the BCAAs and nutrients come from natural, healthy sources. When you train and fuel smart, you get results. Fueling your body with nutrient-rich foods improves your performance. Your physique becomes like that of our ancestors: strong, lean, lithe, and incredibly powerful.

The guidelines we note here aren't enough for endurance athletes. This advise is more for high-intensity exercise that doesn't exceed 60 minutes in duration. If you're interested in fueling for an endurance race or marathon, see the nearby sidebar "Going the distance: Endurance fuel."

Fueling up before exercise

The best advice we can give someone who feels best when eating prior to exercise is to try to eat before that hour window of working out. Eating within an hour before exercising puts you at risk for a *hypoglycemic* (low blood sugar) *reaction,* sometimes called "bonking." This reaction is when you feel shaky, dizzy, and sometimes nauseous during exercise. You want to eat anywhere from one to three hours before you work out if possible. Some people can do pretty well exercising in a fasted state (see Chapter 2), so just play around with different pre-workout timelines to see what works best for you.

Pre-workout foods that tend to work best for most people are proteins and fats. You can keep it super simple and eat any of the following dishes with diced avocado, guacamole, or a nut-based pesto:

✔ Canned fish (check the label for soy)

✔ Leftover meat

✔ Preservative-free and nitrite-free deli meats

✔ Eggs with bacon

✔ Hardboiled eggs

✔ Nuts

✔ Smoked salmon

✔ Bacon and avocado

✔ Olives

✔ Coconut meat, chips, or manna

✔ Nut butter

✔ Shrimp and macadamia nuts

Recovering with post-workout meals and supplements

When refueling after a workout, the key is to eat within 30 minutes after you're done to optimize recovery.

When choosing what to eat post-workout, you want to focus on that fuel called glycogen (see earlier section "Packing a [nutritional] punch with Paleo"). The best way to restock your glycogen stores is through starchy carbohydrates. What (and when) you choose to eat after a workout is your window of opportunity to really gain from your exercise and not be depleted from it.

To rebuild your tissues during this time, you also need those branched-chain amino acids (BCAAs) that we talk about earlier in this chapter; BCAAs are found in protein sources like meat, fish, and seafood. So to rebuild glycogen and rebuild muscle tissues, a meal of protein and a starchy vegetable is perfect. How much you eat depends on how hard you worked and your size. Protein size can be anywhere from 3 to 8 ounces for women and 8 to 12 ounces for men.

For some examples of starchy vegetables, see the earlier section "Vegetables." Berries and dried fruit (in moderation) are also great post-workout food.

Going the distance: Endurance fuel

When you have a race or are involved in endurance training, the trick for fueling before, during, and after exercise is to maintain the right carbohydrate intake for your needs. Figuring out what you need may take some work, but you want to find the balance that restores your muscle glycogen levels and keeps you from bonking.

For endurance training events that last from about 90 minutes up to about 4 hours, you definitely need more carbohydrates before and during exercise. Here, we break down what to eat and when:

✔ **Before exercise:** For best results, eat about 500 to 600 calories no less than two hours before exercise if possible. Your body size, food intake from the day before, and how you feel and tend to trend during endurance races all make a difference. If you eat further in advance (say three hours before), you may need up to 900 calories.

The worst scenario is to eat within the hour before your workout. We recommend eating between two and three hours before if possible and then not eating again until ten minutes before (if you need to). If you eat within that hour window beforehand, you risk having a blood sugar reaction, which may make you dizzy or shaky. However, if you need more fuel, eating again ten minutes before is okay because your body simply doesn't have enough time to pump out insulin before you start exercising, so your body diminishes its need for insulin, and you escape the danger of bonking.

✔ **During exercise:** During exercise, take in 200 to 300 calories per hour. Sports drinks or gels work well here. Solid foods are tough to manage and can even cause nausea.

Make sure you eat or drink from the beginning of your workout, so you don't get in trouble later on when your tank runs low. Drink enough sports drink so you don't get hydrated. Your thirst levels will guide you; just be sure to dial in to avoid dehydration.

Sports drinks definitely have an advantage over water for endurance. Your body turns to protein as an energy source during high-intense workouts, and you don't want your body to turn to protein in your muscles for this. Energy drinks can help your body restore glycogen and, therefore, hold an advantage over water.

✔ **After exercise:** Eating after working out is an important time for recovery. In fact, after exercise is the endurance athletes' most important time to fuel properly. Directly after an endurance race/workout, you need a recovery drink or a meal that contains both carbohydrates and protein in a 5:1 ratio.

For the next few hours, continue to focus your diet on carbohydrates as your body continues to recover. Perfect options are dense carbohydrates, listed earlier in this chapter. For specific meal or snack ideas for recovery, see the earlier section "Recovering with post-workout meals."

Tip: Baby food is great for pre- and post-workout meals because it's easy to travel with and comes pureed so it's also easy to digest. Pick up some protein, fruits, and veggies. If babies eat it, how bad can it be?

Here are some yummy combinations to add into the mix:

- ✔ Eggs, avocado, and blueberries
- ✔ Grass-fed beef over spaghetti squash and sauce
- ✔ Leftover protein and a sweet potato
- ✔ Salads made with protein, jiciama, beets, and carrots
- ✔ Salmon and blueberries
- ✔ Scrambled eggs with diced sweet potatoes (a favorite)

Although nutrient-dense food is always your best support for a healthy body, sometimes you need a little more. If you're in need of supplementation when you make the transition to Paleo to help give you that extra boost, try the following brands, which are some of our favorites, and take as directed on the product label:

- ✔ **Paleologix:** If you need detoxification support, digestive support, or help stabilizing your energy and cravings, try Paleologix supplements (http://paleologix.com).

- ✔ **Primal Fuel:** If you need protein in a pinch for that quick recovery, we recommend Primal Fuel protein powder (http://primalblueprint. com/products/Primal-Fuel.html). It has the healthiest ingredients we have found.

- ✔ **StrongerFasterHealthier:** Taking fish oil rich in omega-3s is great for inflammatory support and for your overall health. StrongerFasterHealthier (www.sfh.com/products) is one of the best brands of fish oil on the market.

Chapter 16

Embracing the Healthy Habits of Paleo Living

In This Chapter

▶ Changing lifestyle habits to get you well and keep you well

▶ Collecting nutrients where you least expect them

▶ Getting the best, cleanest water you can

*N*utrients are essential. Your nutrient levels determine how healthy you are or how open you are to illness; they also affect aging and how well you perform.

When most people hear the word *nutrient,* they think supplements or foods. However, you can make your body healthy, ageless, and strong in other ways. Certain habits provide your body with the nutrition and balance it needs to create a healthy environment and allow your body to flourish.

When you give your body what it needs, it responds by giving you more energy, better sleep, better skin, fewer ailments, and fewer colds and illnesses. You look and feel better all around.

In this chapter, I provide tips on how to give your body the nutrients it needs. I also show you how to get more from your routine through sleep, sunshine, water, managing stress, and Paleo exercise — all of which are a part of truly *living* Paleo.

Making Paleo a Lifestyle

If you want to fully embrace Paleo, you have to *live* Paleo. Living Paleo isn't only about what you do in the kitchen or the gym; it's about the environment you choose to live in. Living Paleo considers how you eat, move, think, and live — it all matters.

When you give your body the right raw material, it flourishes. Giving your body the right food is the foundation, but there's more. You can move yourself toward health by your daily habits — that is, what you *do* as opposed to what you *don't do*.

You can take an active role by making choices that can help your body heal, become strong, and help all the structures and functions of your body work their best. When you map out your day, start looking at some of your habits as ways to give your body that extra burst of nutrition. Sleep, sunshine, water, and stress management are all habits you can use to your benefit to build the best body you can. These simple, free nutrients can make a big difference in your cells and, therefore, in your ability to burn fat, fight aging, get well, and stay well.

Reducing Stress

Almost everything you do rises and falls on how much stress that activity places on your body. In fact, even when you're doing something to boost your immunity, like getting sunshine or exercise, if you get too much, it becomes a stressor to your body and creates havoc rather than health.

Stress comes in many forms, from physical stress to emotional stress. Some stress is short term and can be positive (called *nu stress*) if it gives you that short burst of adrenaline to move you closer to your purpose. The stress that's adverse to your physiology is what's dangerous.

Managing your stress needs to be on your radar. Your body is designed for short spurts of stress, not long-term unrelenting stress. The purpose of your stress response is to get you out of an immediate crisis, like if a tiger was chasing you or you needed to dart away from a moving car. But if your body needs to constantly churn out these stress hormones, you get in trouble fast.

You can relieve stress in a lot of ways. Here are some of our favorite stress busters:

- ✓ **Exercise:** Exercise increases the brain chemicals that make the connections that help you learn better, reverse the aging process, reduce your body fat, improve muscle tone, and also relieve stress. The connections made between nerve cells behave in your body as a natural antidepressant. In fact, exercise is like a natural antidepressant.

- ✓ **Chiropractic:** Chiropractic is primarily aimed at restoring proper spinal mechanics, which in turn influences the function of the nervous system. A properly functioning nervous system is imperative for your cells to communicate properly and for you to feel calm and restored.

✔ **Massage:** Getting a message boosts neurotransmitters *serotonin* and *dopamine,* which are involved in reducing depression and anxiety. Studies even show that your immune system is elevated immediately following a massage.

✔ **The HeartMath Solution:** This program works on what you can do to balance your heart's rhythm, reduce your body's stress hormones, and boost your immunity. For more info, check out the Institute of HeartMath at www.heartmath.org.

✔ **Meditation:** Meditating for 20 minutes twice a day is ideal. If once a day is all you can do, try first thing in the morning while your mind is relaxed. These days, you can use a number of smartphone apps and CDs to guide your meditations in the comfort of your own home.

Want motivation to kick stress to the curb? Stress ages you rapidly. It's also a major contributor to illness, disease, and an unhappy life. Ask yourself these questions before you make any decision: "Is this decision going to add a lot of stress in my life? Is it going to simplify my life or bring complexity to it?" With complexity comes stress. Always have your litmus test ready and ask: "Is it worth it?"

Getting Quality Sleep

Sleep is one of the most powerful tools for health. Think of sleep as the foundation for everything else. When you're deprived of sleep, nothing else you do matters. Your body can't heal and regenerate, and your cells become sluggish.

Sleep deprivation has a pretty powerful overall affect on your body. In fact, when you lack sleep, you risk a lowered immune system, and your number of white blood cells actually decrease. But that's not all. Here are some other potential outcomes of sleep deprivation that may surprise you:

✔ **Illness:** Going to bed too late decreases your immunity and even doubles your risk of breast cancer.

✔ **Weight gain:** You can loose 14.3 pounds a year by getting 1 more hour of sleep a night. (Yes, you read that correctly!) Sleep deprivation causes you to gain weight. Proper sleep helps you lose weight.

✔ **Earlier death:** A 2004 study in the journal *Sleep* found that women who averaged less than 5 hours of sleep per night had a higher death rate than those who slept 7 hours.

✔ **Hormonal shifts:** When you don't get enough sleep, hormones shift, causing your appetite to change. The sugars you crave shoot your insulin up, creating blood sugar problems, weight gain, and health issues.

✔ **Heart disease:** When your hormones shift, causing you to eat more sugar, you get insulin resistance, which causes you to gain weight. During this process, you convert all your carbohydrates into bad cholesterol, and you retain water, which alters your blood pressure. This pattern paves the way to heart disease.

✔ **Altered brain power:** Memory, concentration, and creativity are all impaired with lack of sleep.

✔ **Premature aging:** With a lack of sleep, the body decreases its growth hormone needed for ongoing tissue repair, healing, cell rejuvenation, and bone function. Growth hormone can reverse the effects of aging; therefore, sleep deprivation causes aging.

✔ **Sugar handling problems:** When you're sleep deprived, the ability to metabolize sugar decreases, turning sugar into fat.

✔ **Decreased regenerative powers:** You need sleep to regenerate the body, especially the brain. When you don't have enough sleep, your body doesn't heal or regenerate.

✔ **Prolonged high cortisol levels:** When you're up for long periods of time with the lights on, the stress hormone cortisol doesn't naturally drop like it's supposed to. High cortisol occurs in nature when you need it to run fast or deal with pain from an injury. This constant high cortisol causes people to become panicky and depressive.

Here are some tips to help you make the most out of your shut-eye:

✔ **Go to bed by no later than 10 p.m. and be up by no later than 7 a.m.** Set your phone, watch, or an alarm clock to remind you to close down shop for the night. Most of your body's repairing goes on before 1 a.m., and you get more growth hormone. Your circadian rhythm will also be in sync with your sleep-awake cycle.

✔ **Unplug.** Make sure you're not doing anything but relaxing, journaling, or reading one to two hours before bed. These activities release the hormone melatonin to get you to sleep. That means no TV, no computer, nothing stimulating. Dim the lights if you can to allow your body to start producing even more melatonin. Also move all alarm clocks or electrical devices at least three feet from your bed.

✔ **Black out your bedroom completely.** Your body produces melatonin when it's dark. So cover the windows to prevent any light from coming in. Use blackout shades if you need to. How do you know what's dark enough? When you hold your hand in front of your face, you shouldn't be able to see it. Otherwise, hormone production slows down.

✔ **Keep your room cool and well ventilated.** Keep your room at a temperature that's comfortable for you, but make sure it's on the cooler side. About 68 degrees works for most. Some people also like an air purifier, which can improve the way you breathe and thus improve your sleep.

 Sleep-inducing foods are ironically also powerful immune-building foods. They include foods like turkey, almonds, bananas, spinach, and other leafy greens as well as seasonings and spices like nutmeg, turmeric, and garlic. Calcium and magnesium are also helpful sleep aids.

Soaking in the Sun

Sunshine is like sleep. It's one of those nutrients that people don't think of as a necessity, yet it's imperative to your health and well-being. Just as eating immune-boosting foods are important so is getting some sun exposure.

Soaking up some sunshine is a fantastic way to ward off cancers and other diseases. It also helps your body keep the hormonal rhythm of your natural light-dark cycle. Early morning exposure to sunlight activates your hormones and sets your biological rhythm for the day. This burst of morning sunshine also provides you with a healthy blast of vitamin D.

In the following sections, we outline the benefits of getting a daily dose of sunshine and also explain the best and healthiest ways to expose yourself to the sun's powerful rays.

Realizing the benefits of sun exposure

Everyone knows a good dose of sunshine on a sunny day feels good, but there's also tremendous value to getting some rays. Here are just a few of the fabulous benefits of sunshine:

✔ **Increased immunity:** Exposure to sun increases your vitamin D production, which is an integral part of proper function of the body's T cells, the immune system's first line of defense. Vitamin D decreases your risk of many cancers, colds, and the flu.

✔ **Better sleep:** Exposure to bright light has a positive effect on sleep cycles. Sleep deprivation causes many health problems for which sunshine is protective. Sunshine also regulates the circadian system, which affects sleep.

✔ **Fewer feelings of depression:** A dose of sunlight works magic on depression, especially seasonal affective disorder (SAD). Sunshine also increases the hormones that can affect mood.

✔ **Stronger bones:** Sun exposure gives you more vitamin D and better calcium absorption, therefore, stronger bones.

✔ **Reduced risk of stroke:** Studies show that folks who live in areas with more sun exposure have a lower stroke risk.

✔ **Lower blood pressure:** That warmth that you feel from the sun increases circulation. That, along with increased vitamin D production, is a very affective way to reduce hypertension.

Going in the sun without sunscreen and building a base through slow immersion offers a huge benefit, as we explore in the next section. Through this process, you welcome the production of vitamin D, which helps your body ward off countless diseases, including the following:

✔ Cancer

✔ Diabetes

✔ Heart disease

✔ Hypertension

✔ Multiple sclerosis

✔ Osteoporosis

✔ Psoriasis

✔ Rickets

How much exposure you need to get your dose of vitamin D depends on how dark your skin is and environmental factors (such as how close you live to the equator or what time of day you do your sunbathing). The darker your skin, the more exposure you need. Just underscore in your mind that regular sun exposure is grossly understated as a vitally important barrier to disease. Think of it this way: Regular exposure to the sun protects against skin cancers, and intermittent exposure actually increases your odds.

The benefits of sunshine (UVB exposure) far outweigh any adverse affects. Vitamin D is extremely protective. You can get your levels checked with a simple blood test. In our experience, most people's vitamin D levels are considerably low. So you may need to supplement to "catch you up."

Slowly immersing yourself in sunlight

When it comes to sun exposure, people's fears mostly revolve around sunburn and skin cancer. In an answer to this fear, sunscreen manufacturers promote their sunscreens as protecting against cancer.

The truth is, no evidence shows that sunscreens prevent the main skin cancers: cutaneous melanoma and basal cell carcinoma. Sunscreens protect against sunburn. Sunscreens aren't an anticancer remedy. In fact, because they allow you to have prolonged exposure to the sun, using sunscreens as your only barrier to sun actually gives you a heightened risk of melanoma.

Vitamin D is absolutely one of the most anticancerous types of nutrients your body produces. Blocking UVB really takes away one of the best cancer- and disease-fighting shields your body has to offer.

Intense, infrequent exposure to the sun leading to burning followed by little to no sun actually can cause cancer. These short blasts of sun may cause melanomas and many other cancers. What you don't want, then, is to burn. That strategy is easy enough to implement by practicing the *slow immersion process* — where you gradually expose yourself to the sun over time. When you slowly immerse yourself into the sun, you build a protective layer. Here's how:

- ✔ Build up your tolerance on a regular basis, gradually and early on in the springtime to prep your skin for the stronger sun in the summer. Try to get sun earlier in the morning where you have less chance of burning and overheating.

- ✔ Get frequent short periods of sun exposure, starting with 20 minutes of exposure then building up from there in 15-minute intervals, watching carefully to be sure you don't burn.

When you have to be out in the sun for longer periods of time, and you do need sunscreen, choose one that doesn't contain toxic ingredients. The Environmental Working Group (EWG) is a nonprofit consumer advocacy group that investigates products like sunscreen. It found that many brand-name sunscreens contain unsafe ingredients. So to help consumers select a safe brand, the EWG rated more than 1,700 sunscreen products on the market. Check out the ratings at www.ewg.org/skindeep to ensure that you're using a safe product.

Selecting (And Filtering) Water for Wellness

Your body is made up of about 60 to 70 percent water. Just as your body needs macronutrients (such as healthy proteins, carbohydrates, and fats) to function, it also needs water. Pure, clean water is the most essential of all nutrients. You can live for weeks without consuming food, but you can't go for more than a couple of days without water.

Proper intake of water is so vital to your being that deficiency of even 1 percent can present signs of dysfunctions in your body. Slightly more dehydration, and you get exponentially more health risk.

You also need water to maintain the chemical balances in your body, such as these important functions:

✔ Balancing acid-base levels

✔ Getting nutrients to the cells

✔ Eliminating waste from the lungs, skin, and colon

✔ Regulating hormones

Watch your body's signaling. When you're not feeling well, feeling low energy, or feeling hunger, your first line of defense is always drink water first. Don't let your tank run dry.

In the following sections, we go into detail about the importance of using pure, clean water for both drinking and other household uses. Then we show you how to recognize your thirst signals to make sure you're drinking enough water.

Choosing clean water

When you fill your personal tank with water, you want to drink clean, pure water. You want to create healthy cells, healthy tissues, and healthy surrounding fluid in your body. Clean water helps this process happen naturally. On the other hand, water that has chemicals and toxins can create waste and unhealthy cells.

Having clean water sources in your home is essential. Keep in mind that water that gets into your body doesn't come only from the water you drink; it also comes from all the water sources in your home, like your bath or shower.

You need pure, clean water without chlorine, fluoride, and toxins. The best way to get this kind of water is to install a water filtration system. To make sure you're getting quality water, knowing what's in your water and what needs to be filtered out are good places to start. You can either test the water or at the very least make sure the filtration removes the following:

- ✔ Arsenic
- ✔ Chlorine
- ✔ Chloroform
- ✔ E. coli
- ✔ Fluoride
- ✔ Nitrites and nitrates
- ✔ Parasites
- ✔ Radon

You can choose from a water system that filters the water in one area of your house or one that filters your entire water supply. The best-case scenario is to get the whole-house filtration, which includes bath water, cooking water, and all faucets. What system you go with depends on your personal needs and your budget; just make sure whichever system you choose filters out the chlorine, fluoride, and toxins we list in this section.

Beware of filtered water that's packed in plastic. The chemical bisphenol A (BPA) and phthalates contained in plastics are dangerous to your health. Even low levels of these chemicals cause disease and can create hormonal disturbances. Also, be sure to find out the source of the water you use because 40 percent of bottled water is simply taken from municipal tap water, so most bottled water is nothing more than tap water in toxic bottles.

Watching for your body's thirst signals

People often confuse the signaling in their body. They think they're hungry, but really what they need is water. One of the main problems with this "signal confusion" between thirst and hunger is not understanding how much water you really need and not recognizing the signs of dehydration.

For example, most people wait until they're thirsty to drink. The downside to this habit is that your brain center doesn't send a message that you're thirsty until you're almost 2 percent dehydrated. By then, you've already likely encountered some problems associated with dehydration. Your kidneys receive the low signal before you do, so it responds by decreasing urine output — a big sign that you need more water and fast.

How do you know whether you're dehydrated? The biggest "tell" is if you're not urinating at least six to eight times a day. Also, look at your urine. Is it bright yellow? If so, you need more water. A well-hydrated person has fairly clear to slightly yellow urine.

Following are some ways dehydration plays out in your system:

- Arthritis pain
- Chronic hunger
- Depression
- Excess body weight
- Headaches
- High blood cholesterol
- High blood pressure
- Intestinal pain

Most people have been told that they need about eight cups of water daily. This amount is actually on the low side. You need at the *very least* eight cups. Here's the other surprise: Alcohol, coffee, tea, and other beverages with caffeine don't count as water.

The optimal water intake is half your body weight in ounces. So if you weigh 100 pounds, you need 50 ounces of water daily. When you exercise, you need even more water. Get in the habit of drinking water before, during, and immediately after exercise.

Pre-hydrate in the morning by drinking some water as soon as you get up. Doing so is a good way to get your blood moving and transporting all the good stuff to your body!

Part V
The Part of Tens

the
part of
tens

In this part . . .

✔ Improve your performance when exercising with ten primal superfoods.

✔ Find out how to choose and where to buy Paleo-approved supplements.

Chapter 17

Ten Primal Superfoods to Help You Perform Ten Times Better

*P*rimal superfoods will help get you from where you are now to where you want to be. They have deep nutrition that stand out from the pack of Paleo foods.

Primal superfoods are multitaskers. They heal the gut, decrease inflammation, and flood your cells with nutrients that are often lacking. In fact, superfoods help heal you on the deepest possible level, from the inside out. This healing helps boost your immunity and your energy levels and helps you perform your best.

Push aside your toaster, rice maker, and deep fryer and get ready for some superfoods that will move the needle toward excellence in your physical performance. In this chapter, we list ten superfoods that will make you stronger, heal you faster, and give you a boost toward primal health.

Cage-Free, Organic Eggs

Protein plays a big part in the Paleo athlete's life. Whether you need to pre-fuel with protein and fat or you need to recover with protein and dense carbohydrates, cage-free, organic eggs are your friend. Eggs are a quick protein source that you can have on the ready whenever you need them.

Cage-free, organic eggs are filled with vitamins and minerals, including biotin and choline. Biotin turns what you eat into energy, while choline moves cholesterol through your bloodstream.

Don't put the brakes on eating eggs because you fear the cholesterol. Almost everyone produces less cholesterol in their bodies based on how much they consume in food. Studies show that *dietary* cholesterol doesn't have much effect on *blood* cholesterol.

Fermented Foods

Because your gut has so much to do with your overall health and performance, fermented vegetables (or dairy if tolerated) can be a great part of your food choices. Fermentation uses beneficial bacteria that are great for gut health. Try kimchi or sauerkraut, or ferment some beets or carrots.

If you're one of the few that can tolerate dairy, then fermented dairy is an option as well. Just be sure to choose raw, fermented, full-fat dairy, such as cultured butter, yogurt, kefir, and cheese. You're getting a healthy fat, a fermented food, and conjugated linoleic acid, which has tremendous healing effects.

Full-Fat Coconut Milk

Paleo athletes love full-fat coconut milk because it's high in saturated fatty acids and medium-chain triglycerides (MCT), which are both easily burned as fuel by the body.

Coconut milk is also great to have around and can substitute for heavy cream or yogurt. Buying full fat is important because the lighter versions are simply the full-fat version watered down.

 Always check the labels of full-fat coconut milk and avoid brands with sulfites or added sugar.

Grass-Fed Meats

Getting the right nutrients in your body for a beneficial workout and refueling your body for recovery is critical for success. This is where grass-fed meats really pay off because they're more nutritious than conventionally raised meats.

Grass-fed beef, bison, lamb and goats have less total fat, saturated fat, cholesterol, and calories. They also have more vitamin E, beta carotene, vitamin C, and a number of health-promoting fats, including omega-3 fatty acids and conjugated linoleic acid, or CLA.

CLA may be one of the most potent defenses against cancer. In fact, in a Finnish study, women who had the highest levels of CLA in their diet had a 60 percent lower risk of breast cancer than those with the lowest levels. Switching from grain-fed to grass-fed meat products places women in this lowest risk category. And researcher Tilak Dhiman from Utah State University estimates that you may be able to lower your risk of cancer simply by eating one serving of grass-fed meat each day. You'd have to eat five times that amount of grain-fed to get the same level of protection.

The fat in grass-fed meats are so healthy you can just gnaw on the fat and enjoy — no need to trim the excess fat.

Homemade Bone Broths

Bone broths are flavorful liquids made from boiling animal bones for an extended period of time, often with vegetables or herbs, and then straining out the solids. The resulting broth is rich in vitamins, minerals, antioxidants, and amino acids, which makes you perform your best. Bone broth is a powerful healer that reduces inflammation, heals infection, boosts immunity, stimulates bone health, heals the gut, and even has a calming effect. Check out *Paleo Cookbook For Dummies* (Wiley) for a great recipe for bone broth.

Want to look and feel your best? Add more bone broths to your diet! They heal your gut, strengthen your immune system, make your hair, skin, and nails look amazing, eliminate joint pain, and naturally detox your body. And if you have pets, give them some of this liquid gold for the healthiest coat you can imagine.

Meat Jerky

After you work out, many times you're looking to refuel immediately with a snack. Paleo snacking is different from the modern boxed and packaged snacks. But with a little imagination and willingness to try new things, you can find great options, like meat jerky. The trick is to find a healthy source that doesn't have all the added sugars or processed ingredients. Making your own jerky is another option if you want to avoid added salt or processing and is actually quite simple. Check out any of the many recipes available on the Internet.

Another bonus besides taste is that jerky is a healthy snack you can take on the go. It's convenient and high in protein.

Be sure to purchase meat jerky from the healthiest source you can. Free-range, no antibiotics or added hormones, no nitrates, MSG, soy, gluten, or added sugar. Steve's Paleo Goods is a brand we like; check it out at www.stevespaleogoods.com.

Organ Meats

We know, you're probably thinking, "Why would anyone want to chow down on organ meats?" These meats, which include kidney, liver, and heart, have so much nutrition that it's worth becoming familiar with them. Athletes are always looking for the best sources of protein, and organ meats are definitely one of them. Organ meats have a high concentration of fat-soluble vitamins and are one of the best sources of vitamin D. Organ meats also have essential fatty acids, which are great for your brain and the membrane that lines your cell walls.

The most important thing to know about shopping for organic meats is that quality matters. Getting the finest quality available is essential because not only do organs have deep nutrition, but toxins also store in them. To avoid these toxins, purchase organic, free-range organ meats.

For some really healthy organ meats you can trust, go to U.S. Wellness Meats (www.grasslandbeef.com/StoreFront.bok).

Organic Berries

Organic berries — strawberries, blueberries, blackberries, and raspberries — taste great and are a perfect addition to a post-workout meal. Organic berries are low in fructose (which you want to keep on the low side to avoid blood sugar spikes) and high in antioxidants and nutrition, making berries our favorite fruit. If you can't get them fresh, frozen berries are a great second choice. In fact, having a bag of frozen, unsweetened berries hanging around your freezer at all times is a great idea.

For a super luscious way to eat organic berries, drizzle full-fat coconut milk over them. You'll feel like you're eating a sweet, but because berries are low in natural sugars, they don't create sugar cravings.

Sweet Potatoes

Sweet potatoes take the lead as the number-one recovery food for the Paleo athlete. They give your body the energy you need to refuel and recover. Sweet potatoes are superior to white potatoes because they contain more beta carotene (that's why they have that beautiful orange glow) and contain no antinutrients, whereas the skin of white potatoes do. Antinutrients can cause gut disturbances and nutrients to be depleted from your body, and who wants that? Dice them, sauté them, and mash them with a little cinnamon and nutmeg, and you're set!

Unrefined Coconut Oil

Unrefined coconut oil is our favorite oil to cook with. You can use it for high-heat cooking without making the oil rancid, which can be a big problem. Even if you start out cooking with a healthy oil (like olive oil or macadamia oil), the high heat may oxidize the oil (which means the oil becomes damaged, or rancid), and you end up with an unhealthy oil. When you use unhealthy oils, you create inflammation in the body, which is the back story behind many modern-day diseases, including heart disease.

Unrefined coconut oil is also a good replacement for butter because it's solid at room temperatures and gives you a creamy, delicious taste. It has antibacterial, antiaging and anti-inflammatory properties that boost your immunity for better performance.

Chapter 18

Ten Primal-Approved Supplements for the Modern Man and Woman

. . . .

In This Chapter

▶ Understanding when to supplement and why

▶ Discovering the safest and most effective supplements

. . . .

*T*he cave man didn't have the luxury of supplementation. But it would be downright silly to renounce any and all advancements that have happened over the last million years or so.

Before we go further, we need to make one thing clear: *Supplementation* means "in addition to," not "in replace of." Adding supplementation to a poor diet and exercise routine is like giving glasses to a blind person. It's just not going to do any good. And here's another metaphor: Supplementation is like hot sauce; it can make something that's really good (diet and exercise) even better. And a little bit goes a very long way.

With that being said, not all supplementation is effective or safe. In fact, most supplements out there today are unnecessary and a complete waste of money and time. But in this chapter, we show you ten primal-approved supplements to help you get the most out of Paleo fitness. These ten supplements are actually worth your money.

Creatine

A few years ago, creatine was a hot debate. But the research is now abundantly clear: Not only is creatine safe, but it's also effective. Put your mind at ease because all the myths about creatine being bad for your kidneys have long since been debunked.

Creatine is a naturally occurring acid in your body that helps supply energy, and it's the most commonly used sports performance supplement in the world. It works at the cellular level to replenish your body's primary source of energy, *adenosine triphosphate*. The effect is increased work output.

Perhaps a simpler way to think of creatine is as a stored form of energy that your body can access very quickly. The benefit of this stored energy, naturally, is that it serves to boost your performance in the gym.

Creatine may soon move from being a sports performance supplement to a general health supplement, because it's now showing great promise in preventing and helping treat illnesses, such as the following:

- Congestive heart failure
- Depression
- Diabetes
- Muscle diseases
- Neurological disease
- Parkinson's disease

And if that's not enough, creatine has also demonstrated impressive cognitive benefits, such as the ability to improve memory function and retention.

Is creatine necessary? No, not by any means. And really, if you're following the Paleo diet, you're already getting creatine — because it's found naturally in meat and seafood — just not nearly as much as what's provided in the form of supplementation.

If you think creatine may be right for you, be sure to purchase a form of creatine that isn't tainted with other harmful chemicals (such as artificial sweeteners) or any other unnecessary supplements.

Greens Supplements

Greens supplements are fruits, veggies, grasses, algae, and sometimes grasses that have all been compacted and condensed into powdered form. You can think of greens supplement as the new-age multivitamin. And we actually prefer a greens supplement to a multivitamin because greens supplements come directly from whole, live foods, whereas many multivitamins are synthetic, or man-made. Synthetic multivitamins aren't nearly as potent as a greens supplement, and some evidence suggests that man-made vitamins may actually do more harm than good!

Greens supplements offer a convenient and potent supply of vitamins, minerals, fiber, and phytonutrients, all which help to

- ✔ Boost energy
- ✔ Enhance recovery
- ✔ Improve antioxidant support
- ✔ Support bone health
- ✔ Improve muscle function
- ✔ Reduce inflammation

We recommend that you first try to get vitamins and minerals from whole foods. But we understand that sometimes that can be a difficult thing to do. So a good greens supplement can help fill in the gaps.

When selecting a greens supplement, opt for an organic brand whenever possible and also be sure that it contains no artificial sweeteners or any other man-made chemicals.

Branched-Chain Amino Acids

Branched-chain amino acids (BCAAs) include leucine, isoleucine, and valine and are essential nutrients that the body extracts from protein found in food to build muscle. The term *branched-chain* simply refers to their molecular structure. The most common use of BCAAs for the avid exerciser is to prevent muscle breakdown during exercise and to trigger muscle growth and rejuvenation after exercise.

You may be wondering, "If my body extracts BCAAs from protein, then why can't I just drink a protein shake or eat a high-protein meal after working out?" The answer is that you most certainly could do that. The benefit of BCAAs, however, is that they're metabolized directly in the muscle, whereas other amino acids are metabolized in the liver, which puts them to immediate use.

The added benefit of BCAAs is that they don't seem to instigate any food allergies, like most protein drinks do, making them primal-approved.

Branched-chain amino acids are safe and effective. They're a good fit for anyone looking for a convenient source of pre- and post-workout nutrition.

Fish Oil

Fish oil is good for, well, just about everything and everyone! It's a safe, effective, and primal-approved supplement. Here are just a few of the health benefits that research has linked to fish oil:

- ✔ Improved heart health
- ✔ Relief from depression and anxiety
- ✔ Proper brain and eye development
- ✔ Improved skin complexion (reduces acne)
- ✔ Improved blood circulation

Fish oils contain omega-3 fatty acids like EPA (eicosapentaenoic acid) and DPA (docosahexaenoic acid), which are anti-inflammatory and health-boosting animal fats.

Fish by itself reduces inflammation (which is probably why it helps to alleviate so many problems); this benefit largely comes from its high profile of omega-3 fatty acids. Therefore, regular fish oil supplementation can be quite effective for those who suffer from chronic inflammatory problems.

When selecting fish oil, choose a brand that ensures purity. Although it may cost you a little more, at least you know you aren't taking in any harmful contaminants, such as mercury, arsenic, or lead.

Vitamin D

Unless you spend a great deal of time out in the sun *and* eat plenty of fish, chances are you could benefit from more vitamin D. Vitamin D serves many functions in the human body. For one, it's an immune system regulator and has shown to be useful in preventing illnesses, such as the pesky common cold. Furthermore, research shows that people with adequate levels of vitamin D are at a significantly lower risk for cancer.

Interestingly enough, vitamin D isn't actually a vitamin. Technically, it's a hormone, which explains why vitamin D helps support so many of the body's functions, including the following:

- ✔ Cell formation and longevity
- ✔ Emotional health

✔ Eye health

✔ Heart health

✔ Reproductive health

✔ Skin health

✔ Vascular system health

Vitamin D has actually been shown to help alleviate stress and fight depression. It has also been shown to relieve muscle aches and spasms as well as improve quality of sleep.

Before you supplement with vitamin D, get your levels checked by your doctor to ensure that you take the right dosage.

Probiotics

Probiotics are "good bacteria" that help support your digestive system and overall health. Probiotics work to maintain the natural balance of gut flora in your intestines, which ensures that the digestive system works the way it should.

When the balance of good to bad bacteria in your gut gets out of whack, many problems can arise, including

✔ Bloating

✔ Cramping

✔ Heart disease

✔ Diabetes

✔ Diarrhea

✔ Irritable bowel syndrome

Gut health is enormously important to overall vitality, which is why the Paleo diet focuses so heavily on keeping inflammation low and optimizing the good bacteria in your gut. There's no reason probiotics shouldn't be a part of your diet.

You can get probiotics either in supplement form or through various food sources. For example, kombucha tea is a great source of probiotics, not to mention very refreshing — and Paleo!

Green Tea

Green tea is bursting full of antioxidants, and it's also been shown to have some almost mystical fat-burning powers. In terms of caffeine, green tea is also a lighter alternative to coffee, if you're trying to keep your stimulant usage down — and you *should* be trying to keep your stimulant usage down!

We recommend green tea without any reservations. A cup or two first thing in the morning is a great way to start your day. Green tea is Paleo-approved, and you can have it while fasting, so long as you don't put anything else in it.

Do your best to purchase an organic, full-leaf green tea. Pulverized green tea lacks flavor and potency.

We say *green tea,* but many other wonderful teas are great supplements. Here are a few of our recommendations:

- ✔ Black tea
- ✔ Chamomile tea (a great bedtime tea for its calming effects)
- ✔ Oolong tea
- ✔ Pu-erh tea
- ✔ Red tea (a caffeine-free tea; also known as rooibee red tea)
- ✔ White tea

Coffee

Yes, coffee is Paleo-approved. Really, the only problem with coffee is that people overdo it — and we mean really overdo it!

When we say *coffee,* we mean black coffee. More specifically, we prefer organic black coffee. No sugar. No cream. No syrups. If you're going to put anything in your coffee, try cinnamon or coconut oil.

When consumed in moderation (no more than 2 cups per day), coffee has remarkable health-boosting properties. For once, research shows that moderate coffee consumption may help prevent neurological diseases, such as Alzheimer's.

Furthermore, coffee may actually help strengthen your skin and muscles. Believe it or not, research in muscle biology has found that caffeine stimulates cells in a manner similar to exercise. This doesn't mean that caffeine replaces exercise — no way, no how! — but a little coffee here and there may help you to get more out of your exercise.

Much research has also demonstrated that coffee drinkers are often at a lower risk for certain types of cancer, such as skin cancer, oral cancer, and prostate cancer.

Magnesium

Magnesium is a mineral that assists in nearly all the physiological processes of the body. It's essential and indispensable for proper cell function.

You can get a good amount of magnesium from leafy greens, nuts, and seeds, but as an avid exerciser, you may want to add a magnesium supplement to your diet because it aids in the recovery process. This means that you'll recover more quickly and more efficiently from your intense workout sessions. In other words, you'll get better results, faster.

Other benefits of magnesium include lowering your risk of cardiovascular disease and diabetes, improving the quality of your sleep, and optimizing your hormones.

Whey Protein

Last, but certainly not least, is whey protein. This supplement is a point of contention among Paleo experts because whey protein may aggravate certain food allergies. If you suffer from food allergies, then it's probably best to avoid whey protein. But if you don't have food allergies, then we recommend adding a whey protein supplement to your diet for the following reasons:

- ✔ Whey protein contains a great deal of what's now considered the body's most powerful antioxidant — glutathione. This master antioxidant removes toxins from cells and amplifies the effects of all other antioxidants.

- ✔ Whey protein provides a convenient supply of muscle-building amino acids. If you're a busy person — and who isn't these days? — a whey protein shake is an easy way to make sure you're getting enough protein in your diet.

- ✔ As far as protein goes, whey ranks the highest in terms of bioavailability, which measures how much your body can make use of various protein sources.

The best time to have a serving of whey protein is 30 to 60 minutes after a workout.

When selecting a whey protein source, always be sure to choose a brand that doesn't use any artificial sweeteners or unhealthy oils. To get even more particular, choose a whey protein that's organic and comes from grass-fed cows.

Index

• F •

Notes

Notes

Notes

Notes

Notes

Notes

Notes

Notes

Notes

Notes

Notes

About the Authors

Dr. Kellyann Petrucci earned her bachelor's degree from Temple University, hosted her alma mater's Department of Public Health Intern Program, and mentored students entering the health field. She earned her master's degree from St. Joseph's University and Doctor of Chiropractic degree from Logan College of Chiropractic, where she served as the Postgraduate Chairperson. She enrolled in postgraduate coursework in Europe. She also studied Naturopathic Medicine at the College of Naturopathic Medicine, London. She is one of the few practitioners in the United States certified in Biological Medicine by the esteemed Dr. Thomas Rau, of the Paracelsus Klinik Lustmuhle, Switzerland.

During Dr. Kellyann's many years as a doctor/consultant at her thriving nutrition-based practice in the Philadelphia area, she's helped dozens of patients overcome major health issues while building the strongest, healthiest body possible. With years of research and observation, Dr. Kellyann learned that feeling — and looking — good came down to simple principles and food values that made an astonishing difference in people's lives. Dr. Kellyann found the principles of living Paleo to be the key for those who wished to open the door to losing weight, boosting immunity and fighting aging. With the hundreds of Paleo successes she's seen thus far, Dr. Kellyann is committed more than ever to continuing to spread the Paleo lifestyle message.

Dr. Kellyann has written these health and lifestyle books: *Living Paleo For Dummies, Paleo Cookbook For Dummies,* and *Boost Your Immunity for Dummies* (all from Wiley). She appears on various news streams nationally and conducts workshops and seminars worldwide to help people feel and look their best. She is also the author of the popular website www.drkellyann.com, and gives daily news, tips and inspiration on Twitter @drkellyann.

With her national Paleo door-to-door home delivery food service, www.livingpaleofoods.com, the busy mother of two young sons is committed to making a Paleo lifestyle convenient for everyone, including the extremely busy!

Patrick Flynn is a fitness minimalist, and he wants to help you to eat and exercise more deliberately. Pat believes the secret to a good exercise is simplicity and that any dietary or fitness regimen will improve in direct ratio to the number of things kept out of it that shouldn't be there.

Pat is the founder of ChroniclesOfStrength.com, a top 500 health and wellness blog focused on helping people find clarity in the world of weights through a "less is more" approach to fitness. Pat strips diet and exercise down to its fewest and most fundamental components, helping you to separate the gold from the garbage and to get going with what actually works for forging a leaner, harder, and healthier physique.

Pat writes mostly on minimalistic kettlebell and bodyweight training for strength, mobility, and fat loss. He also covers intermittent fasting, hormone optimization, sex, health, longevity, supplementation, and any other topic that he believes his readers will find somewhat useful.

For a free guide on kettlebell training for strength and fat loss, visit Pat's website at www.chroniclesofstrength.com. Pat also offers private online coaching. It's expensive, but word on the street is that it's worth it.

Dedication

From Dr. Kellyann Petrucci: I dedicate this book to my parents, John and El Petrucci. They set such a high standard for healthy living in my home growing up, and I'm so grateful for that. Now in their late 70s, they are a pure example of the payoff when you chose to live your life physically active, choose to flood your mind with optimism, and are mindful of healthy nutrition. They are as active as anyone in their 40s, and every day still continues to be an adventure. My mother, a beautiful artist, spends her days painting and taking courses from the greatest artist. My father thinks nothing of walking 18 holes on the golf course, carrying his bag with the biggest smile on his face the entire time. Oh, and then there's the "workout." A few times per week, they bust it up in my sister's health center doing metabolic and strength training in the absolute awe of everyone around them. They truly are enjoying their life. All of it.

This attitude does transcend. I would like to think my sister and I (she's a doc as well) have had something to do with their healthy lifestyle, and we certainly have made an impact. But really, it's the other way around. It was my parents' lifestyle practices growing up that made an indelible impression on all of their kids. My sister and I became doctors practicing wellness principles. My younger brother has a black belt in tae kwon do and has been a jujitsu instructor for over 20 years. My older brother is a competitive cyclist in all disciplines and competes throughout the country. He's even a former three-time state champion on the track. We all have taken on healthy lifestyle practices because of the example set before us. Now, all of *our* kids are following the same path. I'm forever grateful I was fortunate enough to have such great role models, whose impact will be felt for generations. Thanks, John and El.

From Patrick Flynn: I would like to dedicate this book to Christine Mooney. I love you. And to bacon.

Authors' Acknowledgments

From Dr. Kellyann Petrucci: I'm super lucky to have Pat Flynn as my coauthor on this project. We first met at a mastermind group and became instant friends. We found that our values and vision for health and wellness were exceedingly congruent and knew this book had to be. I call Pat the "Mark Twain of fitness" because of his great intellect, wit, and charm. These attributes are rounded by the fact that he harbors a unique philosophy on how to exercise and live more deliberately, which makes him the fitness guru to so many. I'm appreciative to have collaborated with him on such a wonderful project and to have become such great friends.

If anyone has ever given you a shot in life, you'll know why I have such deep gratitude for my agent, Bill Gladstone of Waterside Productions. He gave me my first big break purely from instinct, and I am forever thankful for his faith and intuition. Thanks also to Margot Hutchinson of Waterside Productions, who was on my side pitching from the beginning, and who is now more than my agent but a great friend.

To my colleagues at Wiley, especially Acquisitions Editor Tracy Boggier, who has been incredibly responsive and always in my court. To my project editor Tim Gallan, thanks for lending your talents to help us build this book. And big thanks to the masterful copy editor Jennette ElNaggar, who has worked with me on several books and doesn't let me get away with a thing! Thanks.

From Patrick Flynn: The lovely and brilliant Dr. Petrucci deserves my first acknowledgment and by a significant margin. This book would not have been if it weren't for her, and I couldn't have asked for a more capable partner. Her brain is huge, and I wouldn't be surprised if it weighed near to four pounds. Her passion to help others in their quest for health, strength, and longevity is very close to psychotic. And her ability to actually do so is bewildering, if not downright magical. Nonetheless, she is a wonderful woman, charming as a waterfall and overflowing with radiance. Dr. Petrucci, I suspect, knows more about healthy living than the person who invented it, and I would without hesitation entrust to her care my very own sweet and tender grandmother and not have to worry once about phoning for the hearse.

My second acknowledgment goes to that very same sweet and tender grandmother. My third to my mother, fourth to my father, and fifth to my grandfather. (These are in no order of importance, mind you. I'm merely granting them admission as they applied.) My sixth acknowledgment goes to Jennette, the copy editor of this book, for helping me with my spelling and grammar. My seventh acknowledgment I would like to give to my two dogs, Lola and Chewie, who are of the St. Bernard breed and drool quite a bit. I thank you both for teaching me everything I know about quantum mechanics. (And then I said, "That's no St. Bernard; that's my mom!") My next acknowledgment, which I believe brings us to number eight, I give to the whole of The Dragon Gym: Somnath Sikdar, Lonnie Beck, Diana Volante, Chris Taylor, and a few other people here and there whose names and faces escape me at the moment.

My next acknowledgment, my ninth, goes to my agent, Margot. Thank you for selling me. I realize that must have been absurdly difficult.

I am giving my third to last acknowledgment to all my readers and followers over at ChroniclesOfStrength.com. I couldn't do what I do if it wasn't for your kindly donations. (All proceeds, I assure you, go to my direct financial benefit.)

Oh, and my second to last acknowledgment, goes out to the guy who sold me my last car. I think you did a fine job swindling me, and I will find you.

My last acknowledgment goes out to all the rest of my friends in this world. You know who you are, and I will be sending both of you a signed copy of this book.

Publisher's Acknowledgments

Acquisitions Editor: Tracy Boggier

Senior Project Editor: Tim Gallan

Copy Editor: Jennette ElNaggar

Technical Editor: Andrea U-Shi Chang

Art Coordinator: Alicia B. South

Photographer: Rebekah Ulmer

Project Coordinator: Kristie Rees

Cover Image: © Rebekah Ulmer

Apple & Mac

iPad For Dummies,
5th Edition
978-1-118-49823-1

iPhone 5 For Dummies,
6th Edition
978-1-118-35201-4

MacBook For Dummies,
4th Edition
978-1-118-20920-2

OS X Mountain Lion
For Dummies
978-1-118-39418-2

Blogging & Social Media

Facebook For Dummies,
4th Edition
978-1-118-09562-1

Mom Blogging
For Dummies
978-1-118-03843-7

Pinterest For Dummies
978-1-118-32800-2

WordPress For Dummies,
5th Edition
978-1-118-38318-6

Business

Commodities For Dummies,
2nd Edition
978-1-118-01687-9

Investing For Dummies,
6th Edition
978-0-470-90545-6

Personal Finance
For Dummies,
7th Edition
978-1-118-11785-9

QuickBooks 2013
For Dummies
978-1-118-35641-8

Small Business Marketing Kit
For Dummies,
3rd Edition
978-1-118-31183-7

Careers

Job Interviews
For Dummies,
4th Edition
978-1-118-11290-8

Job Searching with
Social Media
For Dummies
978-0-470-93072-4

Personal Branding
For Dummies
978-1-118-11792-7

Resumes For Dummies,
6th Edition
978-0-470-87361-8

Success as a Mediator
For Dummies
978-1-118-07862-4

Diet & Nutrition

Belly Fat Diet For Dummies
978-1-118-34585-6

Eating Clean For Dummies
978-1-118-00013-7

Nutrition For Dummies,
5th Edition
978-0-470-93231-5

Digital Photography

Digital Photography
For Dummies,
7th Edition
978-1-118-09203-3

Digital SLR Cameras &
Photography For Dummies,
4th Edition
978-1-118-14489-3

Photoshop Elements 11
For Dummies
978-1-118-40821-6

Gardening

Herb Gardening
For Dummies,
2nd Edition
978-0-470-61778-6

Vegetable Gardening
For Dummies,
2nd Edition
978-0-470-49870-5

Health

Anti-Inflammation Diet
For Dummies
978-1-118-02381-5

Diabetes For Dummies,
3rd Edition
978-0-470-27086-8

Living Paleo For Dummies
978-1-118-29405-5

Hobbies

Beekeeping
For Dummies
978-0-470-43065-1

eBay For Dummies,
7th Edition
978-1-118-09806-6

Raising Chickens
For Dummies
978-0-470-46544-8

Wine For Dummies,
5th Edition
978-1-118-28872-6

Writing Young Adult Fiction
For Dummies
978-0-470-94954-2

Language &
Foreign Language

500 Spanish Verbs
For Dummies
978-1-118-02382-2

English Grammar
For Dummies,
2nd Edition
978-0-470-54664-2

French All-in One
For Dummies
978-1-118-22815-9

German Essentials
For Dummies
978-1-118-18422-6

Italian For Dummies
2nd Edition
978-1-118-00465-4

Available in print and e-book formats.

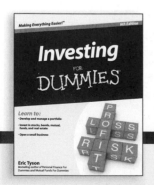

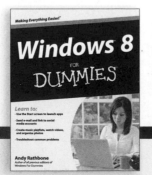

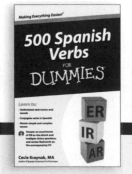

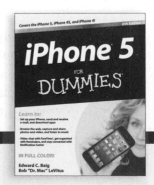

Math & Science

Algebra I For Dummies,
2nd Edition
978-0-470-55964-2

Anatomy and Physiology
For Dummies,
2nd Edition
978-0-470-92326-9

Astronomy For Dummies,
3rd Edition
978-1-118-37697-3

Biology For Dummies,
2nd Edition
978-0-470-59875-7

Chemistry For Dummies,
2nd Edition
978-1-1180-0730-3

Pre-Algebra Essentials
For Dummies
978-0-470-61838-7

Microsoft Office

Excel 2013 For Dummies
978-1-118-51012-4

Office 2013 All-in-One
For Dummies
978-1-118-51636-2

PowerPoint 2013
For Dummies
978-1-118-50253-2

Word 2013 For Dummies
978-1-118-49123-2

Music

Blues Harmonica
For Dummies
978-1-118-25269-7

Guitar For Dummies,
3rd Edition
978-1-118-11554-1

iPod & iTunes
For Dummies,
10th Edition
978-1-118-50864-0

Programming

Android Application
Development For
Dummies, 2nd Edition
978-1-118-38710-8

iOS 6 Application
Development For Dummies
978-1-118-50880-0

Java For Dummies,
5th Edition
978-0-470-37173-2

Religion & Inspiration

The Bible For Dummies
978-0-7645-5296-0

Buddhism For Dummies,
2nd Edition
978-1-118-02379-2

Catholicism For Dummies,
2nd Edition
978-1-118-07778-8

Self-Help & Relationships

Bipolar Disorder
For Dummies,
2nd Edition
978-1-118-33882-7

Meditation For Dummies,
3rd Edition
978-1-118-29144-3

Seniors

Computers For Seniors
For Dummies,
3rd Edition
978-1-118-11553-4

iPad For Seniors
For Dummies,
5th Edition
978-1-118-49708-1

Social Security
For Dummies
978-1-118-20573-0

Smartphones & Tablets

Android Phones
For Dummies
978-1-118-16952-0

Kindle Fire HD
For Dummies
978-1-118-42223-6

NOOK HD For Dummies,
Portable Edition
978-1-118-39498-4

Surface For Dummies
978-1-118-49634-3

Test Prep

ACT For Dummies,
5th Edition
978-1-118-01259-8

ASVAB For Dummies,
3rd Edition
978-0-470-63760-9

GRE For Dummies,
7th Edition
978-0-470-88921-3

Officer Candidate Tests,
For Dummies
978-0-470-59876-4

Physician's Assistant Exam
For Dummies
978-1-118-11556-5

Series 7 Exam
For Dummies
978-0-470-09932-2

Windows 8

Windows 8 For Dummies
978-1-118-13461-0

Windows 8 For Dummies,
Book + DVD Bundle
978-1-118-27167-4

Windows 8 All-in-One
For Dummies
978-1-118-11920-4

Available in print and e-book formats.

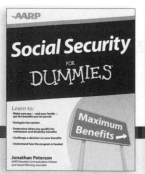

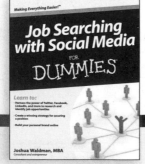

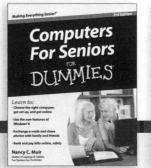

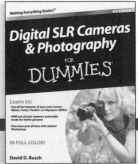

Available wherever books are sold. For more information or to order direct: U.S. customers visit www.Dummies.com or call 1-877-762-2974.
U.K. customers visit www.Wileyeurope.com or call (0) 1243 843291. Canadian customers visit www.Wiley.ca or call 1-800-567-4797.
Connect with us online at www.facebook.com/fordummies or @fordummies

Take Dummies with you everywhere you go!

Whether you're excited about e-books, want more from the web, must have your mobile apps, or swept up in social media, Dummies makes everything easier .

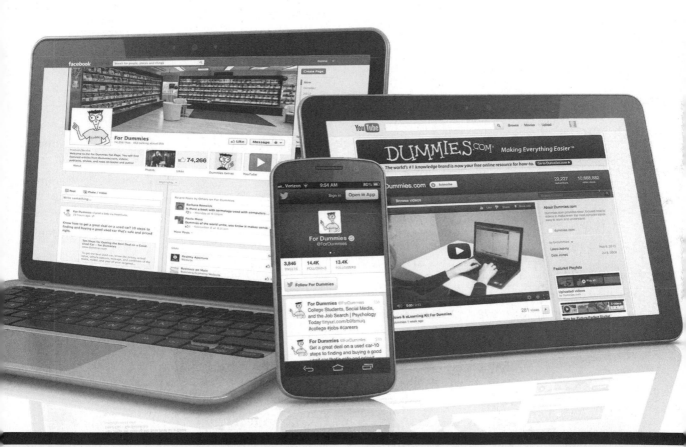

Dummies products make life easier!

- DIY
- Consumer Electronics
- Crafts
- Software
- Cookware
- Hobbies
- Videos
- Music
- Games
- and More!

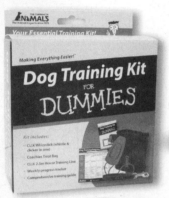

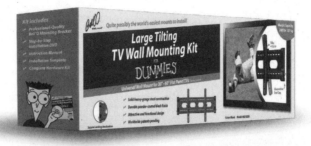

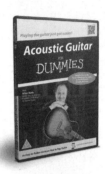

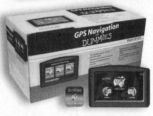

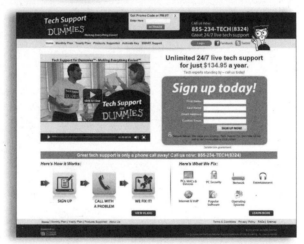

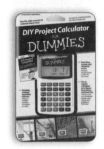

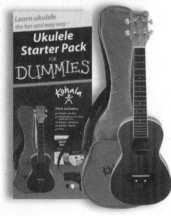

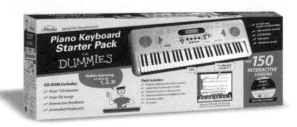

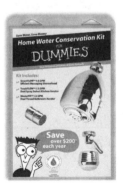

For more information, go to **Dummies.com**® and search the store by category.

FOR
DUMMIES®

A Wiley Brand